It takes a special talent to distill knowledge from an ancient wisdom tradition into a practical guide for a contemporary audience. In *The Kleshas*, Deborah Adele has condensed years of practice, learning and teaching into this down-to-earth, informative, and inspirational book. The personal experiences and the reflections she offers will encourage you to take the lessons off the page and into your everyday life.

~Beth Gibbs, author of *Enlighten Up! Finding Clarity, Contentment and Resilience in a Complicated World*, www.bethgibbs.com

In her new book Deborah Adele offers readers a broad and insightful overview of essential yoga teachings. Along the way she summarizes the classic yoga philosophy of the Indian sage Patanjali, serving up a delightful selection of first hand anecdotes, historical events, conversations, stories, and life as we know it. All this leads to a pathway mirroring ancient wisdom and offering hope to every reader.

~Rolf Sovik, PsyD, Senior Faculty Himalayan Institute, author of *Moving Inward, The Journey to Meditation*

Using a delicate reverse origami of words Deborah Adele does more than 'unpack' the *kleshas*; she reveals them at their most elemental level. In addition to helping us understand the foundation, application, and impact of the *kleshas,* this book also gives us ways to investigate them for ourselves with some suggested reflections and practices. Like *The Yamas & Niyamas*, I'll keep this book at my fingertips to be re-read and savored.

~Kyczy Hawk, E-RYT 500, yoga teacher, writer, and woman in recovery, www.yogarecovery.com

Deborah Adele has a genuine gift for re-presenting ancient teachings in a fresh, accessible way. This new book is an essential text for our modern times—offering an honest inquiry into how our entanglement in the *kleshas* is a root cause of our suffering, and how understanding them can lead us toward transformation. This gives great hope that we all have the power to change and experience the freedom that comes from bringing our scattered minds to stillness.

~Rev. Dr. Sam Boys, Certified Yoga Instructor, Director of Spiritual Life, Culver Academies

This book you have birthed is a remarkable, practical manual for learning to manage our mind and behaviors. Born from the heart of yoga, it offers the modern reader a practical approach for healing our own inner conflicts, and the divisiveness that is tearing at the deep fabric of society. Timeless wisdom presented in relatable, actionable steps that anyone can follow.

~ Sarah Hutchinson R.N., E-RYT 500, Ayurvedic Yoga Educator, www.yogabeyondtheposes.com

The book is so, so good. I love the flow—how you set things up, explain the applicable Sanskrit teaching, add relatable examples, and then break it down further while adding another layer of information. You are especially gifted at relaying lofty yogic wisdom in a way that makes it seem easy! I love that you offer so many powerful opportunities for growth.

~ Sally Burgess, Founder/Owner Studio Gaia Edwardsville, Environmental Activist Illinois Chapter Sierra Club

As a result of her deep inquiry into core human challenges, Deborah Adele makes these concepts come alive as they relate to us in our daily lives.

~Darcy Cunningham, Turning Light Center Founder, www.turninglight.org

THE KLESHAS

A BOOK OF YOGA PHILOSOPHY

THE KLESHAS

EXPLORING THE ELUSIVENESS
OF HAPPINESS

by Deborah Adele

On~Word Bound Books, LLC
innovative publishing ~ Duluth, MN

THE KLESHAS: *EXPLORING THE ELUSIVENESS OF HAPPINESS*
Copyright © 2023 by Deborah Adele

Published by
On-Word Bound Books LLC / Duluth, Minnesota 55812

Fonts
Titling: Benguiat Pro ITC.
Main text: Adobe Caslon Pro.
Poems and call-outs: Rowen Oak by Nick's Fonts.

Works Cited
All direct quotes in this book were reproduced by permission
of the author and/or publishing house. See the Works Cited
page in the Resources section for details.

ISBN-13: 979-8-9867891-0-1

Printed in the United States of America
10 9 8 7 6 5 4 3 2 1

For

Ashly, Tyson, Aryka, Tiana,
Frederick, Franklynn and Lucille

TABLE OF CONTENTS

The goal of yoga is union.
In this union,
the human being is present to the moment,
in sync with what is.
The heartbeat of the human being is
in rhythm with the universal heartbeat.
The limits of the human being are
aligned with the infinite potential of a Higher Reality.

There are no frozen places of past trauma,
no undigested emotional pain,
no mental conflict to interfere with
right action, right feeling, and right thought that
occur naturally from this union.

But this is not the human being
we experience ourselves,
or others, to be.
We are not free of past scars;
we carry emotional hurt close to our hearts, and
we wrestle with conflicting thoughts.

Something is amiss.
For the discipline of yoga,
this "something" is the kleshas.

~ Deborah Adele

Introduction

We want to be happy. We want to feel good. We want our lives to mean something. Yet, happiness seems elusive at best. Sometimes it is unattainable, other times just out of reach. When we do find it, we eventually feel the sting of its impermanence.

Intent on seeking happiness, we find ourselves accompanied by nagging voices of self-doubt, disillusionment, and worry. At times these voices are momentarily silenced; other times they torment us. Something is not right. While seeking to feel good, we experience some form of mild discontent or all out misery. Why? What is it that keeps the happiness and fulfillment we seek so elusive?

Yoga philosophy answers this question in one word: *kleshas*. The *kleshas* form a framework for understanding the discord between our desires and our lived experience. They define the anatomy of what binds us, and they keep us from what we long for. The cause of the discord, according to this philosophy, is a fundamental misunderstanding of who we are, a misunderstanding which in turn cascades into a myriad of misunderstandings causing misery within and around us.

Unaware of the *kleshas,* we continue to ride the waves of life's ups and downs, all the while trying to make the world satisfy our needs for security and happiness. It is as if we go through life seeking, striving, and growing our capacity to have all the things, experiences, and relationships we desire; instead, we become unconscious wardens of our own imprisonment.

Yet the *kleshas* are not all bad news. Understanding what binds us is also what informs us. Knowledge sheds light. When we know how things are, we can make them work for us and eventually, through practice and grace, break free from them, finding the lasting happiness and fulfillment we seek.

The book you hold in your hands is my search for a deeper understanding of the *kleshas*. My focus is on exploring the binding force of the *kleshas* and the practice that frees us from this force. As such, it is not a scholarly commentary, nor does it pretend to be exhaustive in its exploration. It is an attempt to unpack the relevancy of this particular topic in a life as it might be experienced today.

Like the *yamas* and *niyamas*, a description of the *kleshas* is found in chapter two of the Yoga Sutras, authored by the sage Patanjali. Although there is some speculation that Patanjali was a number of contributors or perhaps the name of the school that authored this book, my trips to India to study the Yoga Sutras have shown me a different view of Patanjali than scholarly postulation.

In these settings, Patanjali assumes a role of mythic proportions. Born fully grown, he descended from the sky with a cobra's hood sheltering him, down into his mother's arms. In those quiet studies I participated in in India, Patanjali was invoked with great reverence and devotion, a presence invited to fill the room and teach each of us waiting with open minds and ready hearts. I have sat in the sacred grove in India where Patanjali did his practice and visited the nearby temple built in honor of Patanjali himself.

The Yoga Sutras itself is a unique book if for no other reason than it is the uncontested yoga go-to book. Of all the magnificent ancient texts on yoga and all the current books written on yoga, nothing touches the status of the Yoga Sutras. Made up of 195 short, pithy statements or *sutras*, this is a bold book, an intimate science, a complete step-by-step plan to start where you are and end in the arms of the Divine.

It had to be short because the wisdom was handed down orally. Every word was carefully crafted to explode into timeless, unending wisdom. Disciples would gather at Patanjali's feet to listen to him expand, interpret, and bring to light each verse of the Yoga Sutras. Today we have thick commentaries on this small book to help us unpack the vast knowledge contained in so few words; we could spend our whole lives exploring, reflecting on, and practicing these timeless understandings and their relevancy for our lives.

It is important to note that Patanjali wasn't putting forth a new vision of yoga. Instead, he distilled the experiential wisdom that had preceded him. He synthesized the heart and soul of yoga's timeless tradition. With the authority of those who had gone before him, in conjunction with his own lived experience, Patanjali related the essence of yoga.

In exploring some of these timeless concepts, I have divided this book into four sections. **Section 1, The Problem,** looks at the *kleshas*, the underlying misperceptions of ourselves that we assume to be true. The *kleshas* form a narrative, the conditioning of thought and belief, that is invisible because it is

15

taken as the norm. They limit our happiness, hijack our minds, and promote the very suffering we try so hard to prevent.

I don't start here to be depressive and gloomy, but rather just the opposite. I relish getting at the problem because it gives understanding and guidance, and for me that produces hope. I like to know what is in the way, i.e., what is keeping me from experiencing the fullness of my capabilities. I want to bring the *kleshas* out into the open where they can be seen and examined.

Making visible what has been invisible is often painful, but is also freeing. Knowledge of something previously unknown opens the possibility of scrutiny and choice previously unavailable. It is my hope that understanding our entanglement in the *kleshas* will act as inspiration and incentive to engage in a practice that unbinds our minds and opens us to more than we ever thought possible for ourselves and our world. It is also my hope that we will love ourselves enough to make this effort.

Seeing, as a critical factor in itself, is hard for most of our Western minds. We have been conditioned to fix, analyze, set goals, accomplish…and seeing doesn't feel like we are doing much. Yet as we see, i.e., become aware of, what we have previously not noticed, we gain the power of choice and the desire to engage in a practice that will bring us freedom.

Section 2, The Platform, looks at the mind, how the thinking mind works, and how the *kleshas* interfere with the innate peaceful state of the mind, causing a mind that is scattered, dull, and most often not under our control. The mind is the platform where the battle of bondage to the *kleshas*, or freedom from them, occurs.

Gaining knowledge of the *kleshas* and the role of the mind does not solve the problem of bondage; it helps us understand it. To free ourselves, we need to take action, and for that we turn to **Section 3, The Power**, where we'll explore the process that liberates us from our misunderstanding and places us on the path to lasting happiness and fulfillment.

Section 4, The Peace, looks at what the experience of finding freedom from the *kleshas*, as well as what living with a clear, peaceful mind, begins to look like. What are the lived benefits of freedom on both a personal and collective level? What is on the "other side" of bondage?

Each section of the book is populated with reflection questions. My intention is that these questions support your digestion of the material and deepen the ways you understand the role of the *kleshas* and the importance of practice in your personal life. Reflecting on these questions is a way to take conceptual knowledge into a lived experience. Use them in the way you find helpful.

Writing a book in these times of staggering change, uncertainty, and growing cultural awareness is challenging at best. I am increasingly aware of the "ism's" – sexism, racism, ablism, classism, etc. from which the keen insights of other writers continue to make visible these oppressive "norms." My attempt is not to add to the discussion of any particular "ism," but to explore some of the ways these "ism's" come "ready made" to us, ready to be carried out without thought. My focus is on what is happening in the human mind that seems to accept the status quo of oppression so easily.

I am aware of language and the opportunities and limits that come with it. As more inclusive pronouns insert themselves into awareness, I am choosing to write in the third person "we." I am aware that what I am writing does not always apply to all of us, and that by choosing to use "we," I am also not bringing other pronouns into use. My intention is not to ignore, but to focus on the conditioning itself which undergirds what we accept as the norm.

It seems important to acknowledge that I am writing a book about limited thinking from my own limited thinking, i.e., the limits of my own experience and knowledge. I am white, female, heterosexual, a Midwesterner, middle class, wife, mother, grandmother, in my older years, educated with two masters degrees, and have traveled in Central America, Africa, Europe, and Asia. These give rise to how I see and participate in the world. They also give rise to what I am blind to.

Lastly, I am imbued with a deep belief that by examining the *kleshas*, our children, our earth, the animals, and all those who are forgotten, marginalized, and exploited will not experience further suffering caused from our own failings in reflection, understanding, and discipline.

Kleshas

THE PROBLEM

It is the kleshas that interfere with our experience of happiness, fulfillment, and being in Divine harmony.

What are the Kleshas?

The *kleshas* form a philosophy for understanding the experience of suffering, a term that includes not only external hardship, but the internal suffering of doubt, fear, confusion, worry, disillusionment and feelings of lack. In similar fashion to the Judeo-Christian understanding of being cast from the Garden of Eden, the *kleshas* are an explanation of why human experience is wrought with unpleasantries. It is the *kleshas* that interfere with our experience of happiness, fulfillment, and being in Divine harmony.

Klesha is a Sanskrit word derived from the root word *"klish"* meaning to be tormented or afflicted. There is a progression of five *kleshas*, each giving rise to the one that follows.

> *Avidya* ~ not knowing (ignorant of) who we are
> *Asmita* ~ giving definition to who we think we are
> *Raga* ~ seeking to feel good
> *Dvesha* ~ seeking to avoid feeling bad
> *Abhinivesha* ~ fearing death / loss / change

At the core of it all is *avidya*, the first *klesha*, which is simply that we don't know who we are, and from this fundamental lack of understanding, stem the other four *kleshas*.

The *kleshas* are an acknowledgment that we are born into an inherited world of meaning. Within this framework of meaning, we develop beliefs and habits to explain our unique experiences. We then try to replicate or prevent these beliefs and habits according to our preference. This pulls us into an increasingly solidified pattern that defines our lives by moments of pleasure and moments of pain.

Simply put, the *kleshas* are an understanding of how the story we run in our head keeps us out of harmony with ourselves and the greater whole. It is the *kleshas* that keep us limited and bound and distant to the enlightened state of human wellbeing.

> The *kleshas* are an understanding of how the story we run in our head keeps us out of harmony with ourselves and the greater whole.

None of us set our lives on a course for misery. None of us, when asked what we want for our future would respond, "Gee, I really want to suffer more than anything else." No small child when asked what they want to be when they grow up would answer, "I don't really care as long as I'm really miserable most of the time!" The odd thing is that while we are intent on seeking happiness we embark unwittingly and unknowingly on a path towards increased misery.

It is important to note that the yoga masters did not make this up, but rather watched the normal state of human affairs. Perhaps they wondered why, in this world of abundance and beauty, people experience strife and scarcity. Perhaps they wondered why, when people seek to do things that make them happy, they experience so much unhappiness. Whatever the reason, they observed what happens as humans go about their daily experience. They paid attention to cause and effect. And then they gave voice to what they saw in the philosophy of the *kleshas*.

It is also important to note that by naming what they saw, the yoga masters gave us another way to understand, to expand, and to enjoy the boundaries and particularities from which we engage our individual lives. Understanding the *kleshas* can infuse our lives with enthusiasm and respect. When we see how the *kleshas* work, the world can become a playground of exploration, learning, and vignettes of freedom.

The scholar I. K. Taimni writes, "The philosophy of *Kleshas* is really the foundation of the system of *Yoga* outlined by Patanjali. It is necessary to understand this philosophy thoroughly because it provides a satisfactory answer to the initial and pertinent question, 'Why should we practice *Yoga?*'" (Taimni, pgs. 130-131).

The value of Patanjali's treatise on the *kleshas* is that it shows us where we have unwittingly gone astray. Understanding this philosophy gives us the choice to break free. It is to this understanding of the *kleshas* and their hold over us that we turn our attention.

Avidya ~ NOT KNOWING (IGNORANT OF) WHO WE ARE

Avidya, the first of five *kleshas* and root cause of the *kleshas* that follow, is most often translated as ignorance. Coming from two Sanskrit words, *"vidya,"* meaning "to know or understand" and *"a"* meaning "not," *avidya* refers to "not knowing" or "not understanding" ourselves. We are ignorant of the true nature of ourselves.

It is very strange, I think, to be told we are ignorant of ourselves. We've spent many years being who we are; it's hard to imagine we're anything else. It's hard to feel ignorant when how we know ourselves feels so real.

How is this even possible? How do we find ourselves in a massive state of misunderstanding? What does it mean to be living in ignorance when what we perceive seems clearly real?

There is a consciousness that pervades and undergirds the entirety of all that is seen and unseen. This is our true nature, but it is subtle and quiet. It does not assert itself loudly for our attention. It simply is the essence of all things, including us. But we are drawn to the things that make themselves known through sensory experience. Things like hunger pains, discomfort in the body, and pleasant sensations override the subtle presence of our true nature.

Because the senses are powerful, we tend to know reality by what we can see, feel, taste, smell, and hear. Sensory data becomes our trusted source of information causing us to forget there are other ways of perceiving and understanding or that there might be something more than what the senses reveal.

Not only do we get drawn into favoring the information we receive from the senses, but we are given a conceptual meaning of this information. In other words, we are taught a script of how things are, i.e., a description of our reality. We call this script narrative, conditioning, story, or belief. The thing is, it doesn't feel like a narrative or a story; it feels like reality, and therein lies the problem.

Think of it this way: we were born with limitations. We had no power to physically care for ourselves. It took a few years before we could even recognize a difference between ourselves and our environment. We were born without language. It took time to piece together the sounds of those around us, imitate those sounds, and conceptualize their meaning.

We were born into a narrative that put labels on us, taught us what to value, and told us that the way we see things is the only way to see things.

We were born into a narrative. It was a narrative that gave meaning to who we are, how we are to live, and how the world works. It was a narrative that taught us what to value, what was important, what to think of other people, and how to live our life well. It was a narrative that put labels on us along with the allowed parameters of that label. It was a narrative that told us about God, who God was or wasn't, or even if there was a God.

Most likely we sat on our mother's lap while she read us stories. In these stories, we learned about adventure, friendship, imagination, right and wrong, and emotions such as fear and sadness. Our parents, relatives, siblings, and increasingly our friends became a mirror for us, reflecting back to us our worthiness and value. We learned what was "wrong" with us and how to hide it; we also learned what got us accepted and learned to lead with that.

The stories taught to us weren't taught as one possible way to see things, but as the only way to see things. Rather than being questioned, the stories became the narrative that explained our reality. Thus family, culture, media, education, peers, groups, technology, etc. control the narrative, and thus, the meaning, of our lives. It is from these stories that we learned right & wrong, good & bad, and the shoulds & shouldn'ts of our life.

These stories live in our minds as thoughts, our hearts as feelings and emotions, and our bodies as habitual patterns. They determine what we pay attention to; they determine the mechanisms we employ to cope with the world we live in. They also tell us where we will find meaning, fulfillment, and happiness in our lives. They form the basis for all institutions and laws.

We need meaning. In a world that is unpredictable, we hunger for constancy. Stories fulfill this purpose by giving a stable foundation from which to navigate. But they are a mixed bag. For all they do to provide comfort, security and meaning, they also limit possibility, narrow creativity, and give a reason for violence and hatred.

In his book, *Last Best Hope: America in Crisis and Renewal*, George Packer describes what he calls four narratives that currently exist in America. Referring to these narratives as Free America, Smart America, Real America, and Just America, Packer describes how each of these groups define what freedom means. He goes on to state the importance of each "America" being able to "hear" what is valuable from the others. The book is a hopeful invitation for unity in difference. Yet not many of us are listening to one another, choosing instead to defend our own narrative to the point of incivility and even violence.

Seeing what we expect to see (based on our beliefs) justifies our belief system and catches us in a self-perpetuating feedback loop, reinforcing our own view of reality.

I am reminded of my years as a student of Yogiraj Achala. One of the questions he continuously asked his students was, "What are you not seeing because you are seeing what you are seeing?" His point was always to get us to realize that we see what we expect to see (based on our beliefs), and seeing what we expect to see justifies our belief system. Caught in this feedback loop, our view of reality is not put in doubt.

Today this feedback loop is being solidified in a way never before possible. Behind the scenes of social media and search engines, algorithms are programmed to create a composite of each of us and feed back to us what we like, further validating our perception of reality. On a personal level, our brains and habits are being programmed without our awareness. On a social level, civility, conversation, and compromise are being replaced by polarization, blame, and violence.

Growing up in the 1950's and 60's, we received our news in a very different manner. The news was on three channels (at the same time), lasted for half an hour in the evening, and was very similar in its coverage of the day's events. This meant that those of us watching, from wherever we were, watched the same news. We received the same information, whatever our bias.

This is no longer true. Cable and streaming services have entered the picture and allow for multiple sources of news twenty-four hours a day. Sensationalism has been added to keep us emotionally involved in news coverage. Bots, as part of social media, automatically generate messages, push an agenda, follow other users, and act as their own account. Algorithms are so advanced that if we pause to look at a picture on our feed for the briefest moment, we are "fed" more of the same to hold our interest. The atmosphere is in place for blatant non-truths to parade as truth, truth to appear false, and our minds to be possessed by someone other than ourselves.

It is no secret that we are all biased or that we seek out and enjoy the people who see things the same way we do. Confirmation bias is the word used to describe the phenomenon of constantly seeking and reinforcing what we already "know" is "true." This is the force at work that keeps us from "seeing what we are not seeing."

We need a framework in which to live our lives; we can appreciate this framework because it allows for the stability from which we can co-inhabit this world with other beings. It creates the space for us to expand, grow, and create.

Confirmation bias is the word used to describe the phenomenon of constantly seeking and reinforcing what we already "know" is "true."

But this framework is a limited view of reality; and it is only one of many possible views of reality. As such, it is inevitable that realities differ and often clash. Throughout history, these limitations masquerading as "the reality" have been, and are, the instigators of wars and destruction, as well as order and peace.

Living the limitations and narrative we have been born into is what we call conditioning; mistaking this narrative as "the real deal" is what Patanjali called *avidya*. Seeking fulfillment and happiness within this narrative is the cause of misery; seeking to be free of this narrative is the purpose of a spiritual path.

In the 1998 film *The Truman Show*, Truman is taken as a baby and placed in a limited bubble where he grows up to adulthood. He is content with his life, his wife, his friends, and his job until he begins to notice some peculiar oddities that make no sense. It is not until he risks everything to break free from his town and the life he has known, that he realizes he has been living in a misperception of reality.

For all of us there is a hunger, a drive, a pull toward something more. In *The Yoga Tradition: Its History, Literature, Philosophy and Practice*, Georg Feuerstein speaks to the inbuilt human desire to evolve, a desire he calls the "impulse toward transcendence." This impulse finds many outlets to express itself.

Spiritual traditions understand this impulse as desire, a deep hunger to know and be in full relationship with a Higher Reality, to know who we really are and what we are capable of when we rest fully in our true nature.

But the power of the senses and the framework of our narrative easily pull our desire toward the world, and we find ourselves seeking fulfillment through achievements, possessions, recognition, and relationships. We experience happiness here, but it is fleeting. No matter how hard we try to keep that happiness, it is inevitably followed by loss, failure, and misery. We are powerless to sustain any sense of wellbeing in a world whose very nature is change.

When we are imbued with the knowledge and understanding of the *kleshas*, the world can become a place of enjoyment and liberation. When we look to the world to fulfill us, we are asking the world to give us something it is not capable of giving. We are aware of the desire for happiness and fulfillment, but we are looking in the wrong place. This is *avidya* and it is the cause of the *kleshas* that follow.

It is as if there is a veil hiding the clarity of reality from us, while simultaneously a second veil gives us a picture that we take to be real, and we end up mistaking "the unreal" for the "real." The big questions, "Who am I? Where did I come from? Where do I go? What is the purpose of my life?" all get answered by the narrative. Other possibilities become invisible or simply wrong. Mystery is seemingly solved. Choice is limited.

I attended a lecture given by Pandit Rajmani Tigunait in which he had us close our eyes and put both hands in front of our faces with our fingers on our forehead and the base of our palms on our chins. Then he had us open our eyes and describe our hands. The point is, we couldn't. When we can't see what we can't see, we don't know that we can't see. This is the nature of *avidya*.

We hunger after the possible but fail to ask if it is necessary.

I write at a time when the world is in trouble. We are in the midst of a global pandemic, climate crisis, international discord, civil unrest, racial tension, staggering inequality, and economic disaster. These challenges require us to come together; instead, we are being torn apart by polarities, nationalism, and a failure in self-reflection. The mastery of mind Patanjali writes about seems elusive at best.

We thrive on information but fail at wisdom. We hunger after the possible but fail to ask if it is necessary. We destroy things that feed the soul in order to bring comfort to the body.

For many of us, excess has left us undernourished, greed has left us miserable, disconnection from the earth and the rest of the world has left us lonely, our hectic lifestyles have left us tired and confused, and our growing sense of powerlessness has left us afraid. For many others, lack has produced homelessness, hunger, and a different kind of desperation.

At a time when we need to be awakened from our enamored trance with self, we are being bombarded with messages that support our conditioning and encourage the worst in us. It becomes easy to turn to "them" as the problem and forget to look at ourselves.

Many of us are asking, "How can we turn this thing around?" But perhaps there is a question we need to ask first, and that question is, "How did we get here in the first place?"

"What are we not seeing because we're seeing what we are seeing?"

Questions for Reflection

It is important to note that the yoga masters were avid observers of the way things are. They watched and paid attention and then gave explanation to what they saw and experienced. They saw with the eyes of curiosity, not the eyes of "right and wrong" or "good and bad." They simply wanted to know how things worked; what caused what.

As you reflect on *avidya* and the questions below, take the stance of seeing how things are without judging them. The *kleshas* are not good or bad in themselves, they are an explanation of how things are.

Reflection: What are some of the things that shaped you growing up? What did your parents (or caregivers) ingrain in you? Were there any particular television commercials or shows that influenced the way you saw yourself and the world? What about songs? Books? Friends? School? How were these things beneficial? How did they limit you?

Reflection: Name a culture very different from your own. Name something you find odd about this culture's beliefs or customs. Would you find that thing normal if you had been raised in that culture? What about your culture might someone from that culture find odd?

Reflection: Explore Yogiraj Achala's question, "What are you not seeing because you are seeing what you are seeing?" What is your experience of asking this question? What is your experience of answering it?

Reflection: Describe your experience of what Georg Feuerstein calls "the impulse to transcend." Do you feel it as a gnawing sensation, a hunger to know, a desire to have, a drive to achieve, a need for more, or......? How do you try to fulfill this feeling?

Asmita ~ GIVING DEFINITION TO WHO WE THINK WE ARE

Because we don't understand our true nature, we identify with what we do know about ourselves and call that "me." Thus *avidya* gives rise to the second *klesha*, *asmita*, a sense of "I-ness" that is identified with our experience in the world.

We could think of *asmita* as ego, and for all practical purposes it is, but there is a differentiating quality. Ego is the process that makes us feel separate (in the next section on the mind we will look at this separating process in greater detail). *Asmita* is the specific roles, talents, personality, etc. we identify as ourselves.

Thus we know ourselves not only as a separate entity, but with specific qualities to that separateness. We know ourselves as our roles, successes, failures, achievements, regrets, feelings, thoughts, and moods. We know ourselves as our gender, sexual orientation, skin color, nationality, and class. We know ourselves by the value and parameters placed on us by the culture we live in. We know ourselves by how we see ourselves fitting in the world and by how we think others see us.

The way we learn to know ourselves does not come from our own inner passion and deep awareness. Instead, it comes from others' naming of us. We hear over and over that we are the smart one, the successful one, the funny one, the rock that holds everyone together, or we are the big disappointment. As Pandit Rajmani Tigunait once said in a lecture, it's as if others put stickers on us and we believe we are what the stickers say about us.

When I was young, I enjoyed playing with paper dolls. The dolls were made of cardboard and came with stands to keep them upright. A variety of outfits came with the doll. Each outfit had a crucial number of small tabs that would bend to attach over the doll. In much the same way, *asmita* is like dressing paper dolls. We put a story over our experience and interpret the experience through the story. We remember ourselves more than we experience ourselves. One difficult event defines us; disease defines us; unworthiness defines us; victimhood defines us; success defines us. We are limited by the stories we tell and the behavior that is associated with these stories; it is difficult to see ourselves in any other way.

> As we wear the identity placed on us, we identify with it so strongly that we tend to hear only what reinforces this sense of self.

As we wear the identity placed on us, we identify with it so strongly that we tend to hear only what reinforces this sense of self. At the same time, we are deaf to words and experiences that tell us something different about ourselves. This process, referred to as the flypaper/Teflon process, means we stick like flypaper to words and experiences that reinforce our sense of self. Anything contrary to our self-identity has no sticking power; it slides off our psyche like food slides off a Teflon pan.

We believe that success looks a certain way (the way culture tells us it looks). If we meet this standard, we are successful; if we don't meet it, we experience ourselves as a failure. The same is true for standards of beauty. Not only is our identity wrapped up in the narrative's standard, but how we compare ourselves to that standard determines our sense of self-worth. If we do not question the standard, we have to shrink our own valid experience so it will somehow fit into the narrative, even if it means demeaning ourselves.

Or we may become rebellious, relishing the fact that we are not willing to conform. If we look closely, however, we find that rebellion is often an opposite reaction to the norm; it is not a transformative process. Either way, we are formed by what we are told.

In a particular class I was teaching, I asked participants to make a timeline of the statements that shaped them. They were to note the age they were, where the influential statement came from, and any historical events of the time. Then they were to get into small groups and discuss what they had sketched out on paper. One group consisted of two women, both named Mary. They were about the same age, had similar backgrounds and experiences, and each had a sister. The defining difference in the shaping of each of their lives came from their mother. One Mary was consistently told, "Why can't you be more like your sister?" The other Mary was told, "Whatever you do, don't be like your sister!"

Believing ourselves to be a certain way puts pressure on us to show up that way. It also means we are training others to see us the way we want them to. If we are the "funny one" or the "one that can always be counted on," then we always have to be funny or be there for others. The pressure to "be that way" results in the eventual need to lash out at others for expecting so much from us or to chastise ourselves for our failure to meet those expectations.

> Believing ourselves to be a certain way puts pressure on us to show up that way. It also means we are training others to see us the way we want them to.

The bottom line is that we spend our energy trying to elicit approval within the standards that have been imposed on us and that we have imposed upon ourselves. There is always something to do, something to attain, something to protect, and something to fear in order to get and maintain this approval.

After the publication of *The Yamas & Niyamas: Exploring Yoga's Ethical Practice*, I had several opportunities for interviews. During my first interview, I was asked, among other things, what books I read before going to sleep. I answered that I read the mystics because I wanted to feed my soul.

Later that evening when my spouse came home, we listened to the entire interview. When I was asked the question about what I read at night, my spouse and I, upon hearing my response that I read the mystics, looked at each other and burst out laughing. My response was a lie; at the time of the interview, I played Sudoku before I went to sleep.

An even bigger shock was not only had I lied (on my first interview after writing a book on ethics), but I didn't know I had lied until I heard myself! I was beyond horrified. Upon reflection, I realized that I had fallen victim to an image of who I thought I should be now that I was a yoga studio owner and an author of a book on ethics. I had answered according to my perceived image.

Almost a decade later, I am still horrified by this event and certainly humbled by it. It was truly an experience of the power of *asmita* to control my sense of self to the point of deception.

Asmita not only elucidates the definition and standards that bind us, it dictates what we see as acceptable behavior in others. From our partner and friends, to people we don't know, we "reward" them with our approval if they behave in the way we think they should. If they don't behave that way, we can find ourselves withholding approval in various subtle or not so subtle ways.

People who are "not like us" receive the brunt of our inability to look honestly at our own conditioning and beliefs. Oppression, rudeness, scorn, unequal opportunities, slanted justice, brutality, murder, and genocide are the lived reality of our preference to believe lies and scapegoat others, rather than ask ourselves hard questions.

With family members and friends, we speak too easily about what "someone else has done," not realizing that we do it quite consistently ourselves. Our annoyance with others betrays our own inability to grasp the truth of ourselves.

We also project our courage, leadership abilities, and vision onto others. When we give these things away, we impoverish the world by not showing up in our full capacity. Not developing and sharing the talents we were born with is a sure way to cheat the future. And yet the psychological mechanisms we have in place for protecting these virtuous and not so virtuous parts of ourselves don't allow us to see ourselves accurately.

The structure of *asmita* defines what is possible, and it does this by offering limited options that pretend to be freedom of choice. In the world my mother grew up in, two options existed for her. One was to become a teacher, the other a secretary. What looked like a choice my mother got to make was a narrative that restricted her options. It takes time before someone begins to question the limits of the choices themselves, and then it takes the efforts of many for the narrative to change.

> Our annoyance with others betrays our own inability to grasp the truth of ourselves. We also project our courage, leadership abilities, and vision onto others. When we give these things away, we impoverish the world by not showing up in our full capacity.

Yogiraj Achala used to explain the process of limits using the analogy of snow. "It's all snow," he would say, "This creative power of consciousness goes about making snow men, snow women, snow villages, snow cars, etc." The problem comes when we lose sight of consciousness and take all of these creations as separate entities, including ourselves. Instead of identifying with snow, we identify with all the things that snow takes the form of.

As our identification with form solidifies, our basic biological needs get tangled up with our conditioning. As biological beings, we have needs that must be met in order to survive, and we have instincts to sound an alarm when those needs are in jeopardy. Instincts are there to keep us alive and flourishing, and under ideal circumstances they function naturally. We feel hunger and reach for food that is good for us and in the correct amount. There is an appropriate response to the instinct.

But when the instincts run through the conditioning of the narrative, they can easily get distorted. From the viewpoint of *asmita*, our needs can feel threatened. For instance, our hunger, instead of being simply satisfied, can become anxiety about not having enough food or not being good enough. We can find ourselves reacting to this anxiety by overeating, eating sugary treats, and/or hoarding food. The conditioning of *asmita* hijacks the instincts and they begin to serve *asmita's* story, rather than the basic needs of the organism. In allegiance to our sense of "I-ness," they feel non-negotiable.

And so we worry, we fret, we fear. We focus on ourselves and become selfish, greedy, judgmental, even hateful. We allow painful things to happen to others so that we can feel protected and secure. We find ourselves wondering, "What possessed me to do that?" when instincts, at the mercy of conditioning, override our sensibility. Self-interest and fear distort our physical welfare and our relationships.

We are almost always experiencing some form of conflict between living the narrative expected of us and following the inner pulse to know our full self. We feel this conflict in various ways: as doubting our inner voice, as living the "shoulds" of our life, as scoldings from the inner critic, as feelings of guilt or shame, as feelings of unworthiness, as "shrinking" ourselves to "fit" the narrative, as turning to addictive habits, as squelching our creative force, as losing our vitality.

In 2019 I broke my arm while hiking. It was a hard fall, which displaced the fractured bone, and resulted in surgery. Having never broken a bone, I expected after many weeks of wearing a cast that my arm and hand would function as usual. I was surprised when my expectation proved false. My elbow was stuck in a 90 degree angle. It had forgotten how to straighten. My wrist had forgotten how to rotate. My fingers had forgotten how to extend or curl. My arm had forgotten how to be an arm!

This is much like what happens to us in *asmita*. The descriptions and roles we identify as "us" are like a cast. As we continue to identify ourselves with the descriptions and roles, we become more defined by them. We get more interested in trying to make our identity "work" than in asking the bigger question, "Who am I really?" Our reality shrinks; we shrink. Without a new way to see ourselves, we become further entangled in the *kleshas* that follow.

Questions for Reflection

We are spiritual beings having a human experience, and having a human experience is limiting. These limits are neither good nor bad in themselves; they simply are the way things are. But who defines those limits for us? What do we believe about ourselves and where did those beliefs come from?

Reflection: What are the "stickers" others have put on you? What are the "stickers" you have stuck on yourself? What are the stories you tell yourself about yourself?

Reflection: Notice the voice of your inner critic and how it is the police force for your identity narrative. What does your inner critic say to keep you "in line" (i.e. in line with the story of who you should be)? How does this voice make you feel? Now notice the voice of your inner knowing. What does the voice of your inner knowing say to you? How does this voice make you feel? Which voice are you most likely to listen to? Why?

Reflection: Notice how you think you are your thoughts and how you believe what your thoughts tell you. What do your thoughts have to do with you and how you perceive yourself?

Reflection: Notice places in your life where your instincts (for basic survival necessities) get hijacked by your conditioning and lead to inappropriate, unnecessary, or even harmful actions.

Raga ~ SEEKING TO FEEL GOOD

From the time we are born, we know pleasure and pain.
We feel the pangs of hunger in an empty stomach. We feel
the discomfort of wet, dirty diapers. We sense the fear of
being abandoned or the insecurity of being carelessly held.
Likewise, we feel the pleasure of sucking warm milk and
feeling it fill our tummies. We feel the joy of being cooed
at, admired, and loved. We learn to love the attention and
approval of others and the sense of satisfaction in our being.
We learn to want more of this pleasure and avoid as much
discomfort as we can.

Our desire to experience pleasure is natural; it is our innate
state to be happy. But *avidya* and *asmita* have us so entangled
in the outer world that we end up seeking happiness outside
ourselves. This dependency on the outer world to make us
happy is called *raga*, an attachment to the people, objects, and
experiences that make us feel good.

One of the tools that guides us in our search for pleasure is
memory. We remember how good we felt when we were with
a particular person. We remember the delight we experienced
when we ate a certain food. We remember the excitement of
participating in a particular event. We seek the experience of
happiness, and our memory reminds us where that happiness
can be found.

My spouse and I speak on the phone regularly and often ask
each other how our day is going. As I began to wonder what
was behind my answer, I realized my response was dependent

on things going my way. If my expectations were being met, it was a good day. If my expectations were being surpassed, it was a great day!

We could think of *raga* as our personal agenda for happiness. Fulfilling this quest demands the bulk of our attention and focus. It consumes our energy. It sets up expectations on others. It solidifies our habits and thought patterns. It deepens our dependency on what is outside ourselves. Unwittingly we use manipulation and control, trying to make things happen that are beyond our power to do.

We become slaves to the perfect latte, lights that turn green as we drive down the street, our living space exactly the way we want it, and our significant others, children, bosses, and friends to be easy and accommodating. Whether consciously or unconsciously, we demand that everything and everyone be responsible for our happiness.

> Memory creates the expectation that the repetition of a previous event will make us happy like it did before.

The memory of finding happiness where we found it before creates the expectation that we will find it there again. Said another way, memory creates the expectation that the repetition of a previous event will once again make us happy like it did before. It doesn't take much to see this is a plan doomed to fail. Each successive chai we order needs to be better. Each time we are with our friend, the experience needs to be more fun or more intimate. *Raga* thrives on our desire to have more. The stakes get higher as the need and expectation keep rising.

Without awareness, our actions become repetitious. We cling to our habits, even if they aren't always effective. We do more of the same, hoping this time we will get a favorable result. We turn to outside sources to understand what we are doing wrong. Although these sources can be helpful in guiding our inner wisdom; they are dangerous when we give them power to be the magic bullet that unlocks the secret to constant happiness.

Our behavior becomes a frantic, mostly unconscious crusade for demanding that the things of the world meet our expectations to make us feel happy. We become confused at why it isn't working, and, instead of reflecting on the situation, we try harder. We can even do this to our yoga practice, or any spiritual practice, demanding that it brings a steady dose of happiness to our lives.

To make matters worse, there is an emotional component to attachment. One would think that when things are going our way, we would become a more pleasant person. But that isn't necessarily true. Although we may seem pleasant for a while, underneath, vices are being fed. Pride is strengthened as we give ourselves credit for our good fortune. Greed ramps up its insatiable demands. And as we become increasingly dependent on this person or that thing to make us happy, attachment grows.

When we are expecting something to make us happy and it

doesn't, disappointment creates strong reactive emotions. We feel anger, even rage, because we didn't get what we wanted. We also feel envy as we look around and see that others have what we want; it's just not fair that they have it and we don't.

Emotions bring a visceral, skin in the game, sense to our experience. By adding a feeling component, emotions solidify our conditioning and further compromise our clarity and common sense. As a result, ego grows more demanding and rigid, and *raga* continues to consume us in a fruitless search for lasting happiness.

This search in the outer world for happiness often confuses our sense of what is really important. A friend of mine who loved motorcycles bought a vintage Italian one for his wife. On a road trip together, she had an accident. Both she and the motorcycle were lying sprawled on the road. My friend went to the motorcycle first to see if it was okay and left his wife lying there. He had more angst over the machine than his living, breathing partner, and she never forgave him.

In another incident, an acquaintance told me about buying a cat because he wanted to have something to snuggle with while he watched television. The problem was, he reported, that the cat he purchased didn't like to cuddle or even sit on his lap. The person was so put out with the situation that he threw the cat outside the house and never cared for it. The sole reason for purchasing the cat was to fulfill a personal need for pleasure. When the cat failed to make its owner "happy," the cat was thrown out to fend for itself.

The levels of cruelty in this story are the result of *raga*. The person in the story had no thought for the cat's wellbeing. He had no sense of responsibility to this living creature. He only wanted the cat to fulfill his own desire for pleasure. And when the cat failed to give that pleasure, the cat was simply dismissed. This is but one example of how *raga* distorts our priorities and compromises our humanity.

> There is nothing wrong with enjoying pleasurable things or having preferences. The problem comes when we cling to our personal pleasure list, demanding that it happen on our terms and meet our expectations.

As we consider the cruel places that *raga* can take us, it is valuable to remember that pleasure and enjoyment are not the problem; nor is having preferences. There is nothing wrong with enjoying pleasurable things; there is nothing wrong with having preferences. In fact, the yoga masters teach us that life is for our enjoyment as well as our liberation. The problem comes when we cling to our personal pleasure list, demanding that it happen on our terms and meet our expectations.

If we can open ourselves to find contentment when we receive what we want as well as when we don't, we may find ourselves enjoying things that used to annoy us. If we continue to cling to our personal list, we move deeper into entanglement with the next *klesha*.

Questions for Reflection

As you reflect on *raga* and the questions below, remember to watch the process of your pleasure seeking, not judge it. When we judge ourselves and our actions too quickly, we miss the importance of the process itself. For now, watch how much of your orientation is towards the things that give you pleasure and the ways you define pleasure (pleasure for you will be different than pleasure for someone else). Notice what you do to get pleasure. Feel and sense in your body and nervous system what is happening as you move towards something and cling to it. Remember, we are trying to know ourselves, not fix ourselves.

Reflection: What is your personal agenda for happiness? In other words, what needs to be happening outside yourself for you to feel happy inside? Where did this agenda come from?

Reflection: Notice ways you attempt to control or manipulate each moment to get what you want (or to keep it). Pay attention to the emotional factor that goes with the results of your efforts.

Reflection: Can you enjoy your life without the need to have it on your terms? Do you really need things your own way all the time?

Reflection: Have you ever sacrificed your integrity (even a little) to get what you wanted? What were the end results? How did it make you feel?

Dvesha ~ SEEKING TO AVOID FEELING BAD

Dvesha is the avoidance of that which causes pain or puts our pleasure at risk. Commentaries use the word aversion, pain, or repulsion to translate this *klesha*. Coupled with *raga*, our pleasure seeking tendency, *dvesha* sets up a deepening requirement that life happen on our terms.

As noted earlier, it is our innate state to be happy so it makes perfect sense that we would want to avoid anything that interferes with our happiness. We avoid loud noise because it threatens our preference for quiet. We avoid being alone because we love how we feel surrounded by people. We avoid cold climates because we prefer warmth.

As with attachment, it is desire informed by conditioning and memory that defines avoidance. We remember a particular person, object, food, or event caused previous displeasure. The memory of previous displeasure causes our psyche to contract, recoiling from just the thought.

Unpleasant memories require us to maintain a hypervigilant state, always on the lookout to prevent an unpleasant experience from repeating itself in the future. This kind of vigilance against the unpleasant produces an undercurrent of anxiety and worry that becomes our constant companion.

This is not to say that vigilance is a negative word. Responsibility to our young children requires a certain attention to their safety. Responsibility to driving a vehicle requires a certain attention to motor signs as well as to other drivers and pedestrians. Rather, the vigilance caused by *dvesha* is in service to our personal agenda, not to our responsibility as a human being.

Dvesha happens with the memory of an unpleasant or painful experience or from the experience itself. It happens when we can't make a pleasant experience happen or when something puts the pleasant experience at risk. It happens when we are at the mercy of a trauma experience. Physically, we experience *dvesha* as contraction, repulsion, or resistance. Emotionally, we experience *dvesha* as misery, disappointment, frustration, irritation, blame, or anger. We can viscerally feel this tightness grip our psyche and keep our nervous system on edge.

Dvesha can happen in petty ways. Someone hurt our feelings, so we stop going to the places where we might encounter them. We were served a disappointing meal at a restaurant, so we stop frequenting that restaurant. Our sibling says something we don't agree with, so we refuse to be in the same room with them. As more and more things displease us, our world becomes smaller. And the more we entertain the thoughts of the unpleasant experience, the more negative our mind becomes.

If *raga* can be thought of as the need to fulfill our personal agenda for happiness, *dvesha* can be thought of as the need to accommodate our weaknesses. *Dvesha* demands we cater to our conditioning rather than break free of it. Instead of developing our patience and tolerance, we weaken our character by making sure nothing we dislike happens to us. Think about how small *dvesha* makes us. Rather than staying curious and open, our attention is turned towards making sure nothing unpleasant, large or small, happens to us.

The shrinking path of *dvesha* can be oddly distorted. We can come to enjoy the attention we are receiving from our illness so much that we avoid healing. We can come to enjoy the sympathy we receive from a miserable situation so much that we avoid changing it.

At the height of a pleasurable experience, we can find ourselves recoiling at the thought of the experience ending. We can have so much enjoyment with someone that the thought of losing them makes the pleasurable experience simultaneously painful.

We can avoid making connections. Even if we believe in climate crisis, we won't let ourselves make the connection to how much gas we use. Even if we know women suffer in sweatshops, we won't let ourselves make the connection to a cute red top that we just have to have. When these truths put our pleasure at risk, we avoid facing them. We avoid being inconvenienced.

Pandit Rajmani Tigunait points out the danger of this *klesha* when he says, "*Dvesha* is a condition of the mind that has no tolerance for an enemy." He goes on to say, "We deny we are possessed by hatred and instead claim to hate only a particular person or circumstance. We insist there is a good reason for this. In short, we rationalize our hatred, anger, vengeance, and violence" (Tigunait, p. 52).

How many times do we hear ourselves or someone else say, "That person makes me so mad!" This is Pandit Rajamani's point. When someone puts our pleasure at risk, it gives us a place to hang our hatred and then feel justified because "they" made us feel this way! It's a brilliant move by our egos. We get to feel justifiably put out (because our preferences were interfered with) and excused from looking at the hatred that sits inside of us.

Countless times I have asked my spouse to do a chore. I notice when he doesn't do it the way I want it done, I feel irritated with him for not doing it right. The truth is, the irritation sits in me waiting for someone to blame when things don't happen to my preference. I have conveniently deposited my own shortcomings on him, rather than taking responsibility for the weakness that sits in my own psyche.

The above scenario can be a cause of strife in our relationship. The years spent together have grown a loving acceptance of each other, so the strife is felt more as a subtle undercurrent of unrest, rather than as open bickering. But as long as I need things my way, and he needs things his way, some form of unrest remains intact. And we are each conveniently able to blame the other for the unrest.

Our propensity to project blame at the group level when our preferences are thwarted, often leads to war, genocide, and other forms of mass atrocity. Our ability to put our own failings outside of ourselves allows us to dehumanize the other, while feeling self-righteously justified. From this place, we are capable of causing great harm. To repeat what Pandit Rajmani Tigunait says, "*Dvesha* is a condition of the mind that has no tolerance for an enemy" (Tigunait, p. 52).

> Our propensity to project blame at the group level when our preferences are thwarted, often leads to war, genocide, and other forms of mass atrocity.

The two *kleshas*, *raga* and *dvesha*, are a dynamic duo that work seamlessly together. Our experience is quickly categorized into pleasure/pain, attachment/avoidance, like/dislike. Our bodies react with a pulling/pushing, clinging/recoiling response. Our mind is in a constant turbulent state of oscillation. Our emotions fluctuate from high to low. Our psyches are exhausted. We have become prisoners to our own likes and dislikes.

We savor aromas that please us and hold our nose when we find them disgusting. We light up when our neighbors fit our picture of what a good neighbor should be, and we place unkind judgments on the neighbors that fail to meet our standards. We place an adjective or adverb on every person, thing, or experience we encounter, categorizing everything into a like or dislike.

This all feels real to us because it is such a visceral, lived experience. Where *asmita* wrapped our sense of self in a limiting narrative, *raga* and *dvesha* further drag our sense of self into identifying with the desire we are feeling, along with the person or object of our desire. When that desire is met, we feel happy; when it isn't, we feel angry...and we think it is all due to that particular person or object.

Rather than taking responsibility for our own weaknesses, or our own wellbeing, we conveniently place them on a person or object outside ourselves.

One evening when I returned home from teaching, I was surprised to find my spouse had picked up the house, done the dishes, and told me how beautiful I was when I walked in the door. I watched myself feel a great deal of pleasurable satisfaction, followed by the thought that this kind of homecoming was rare, which made me sad. Then I watched myself try to figure out how to hold on to this experience or at least have it repeat itself every night. The mental gymnastics ended in failure and the experience waned as the evening progressed. In split seconds I rode the waves of pleasure/pain and all the thoughts and feelings that accompanied it. My physical, mental, and emotional states were at the mercy of my likes and dislikes and all because of one extra pleasurable experience.

I remember sitting on a small rug on the ground at an ashram in Santosh Puri, India. The sun was hot and the flies were buzzing. Along with other students from various countries, I was listening to Mataji (Narvada Puri) speak her wisdom gained from years of study and practice. This particular time she was more animated than usual as she tried to awaken us students from our entanglement in our likes and dislikes. With voice raised she proclaimed, "You Westerners, you think if you do things right life will always go the way you want it to. Don't you realize life is like a quarter that consists of heads and tails? Life brings waves of ups and downs. You need to stop riding the waves and stay established." In my mind I can still see the passionate gestures that accompanied her words, one hand going up and down, the other moving in a straight line. She was demonstrating the power of staying established in equanimity no matter what is occurring around us.

As our sense of self becomes wrapped up in our attachments and avoidances, we forget to wonder where our preferences came from and why they have so much control over us. We forget to ponder if there might be more meaning to our lives than getting what we want. We fail to notice how small our world is becoming.

56

Questions for Reflection

As you reflect on *dvesha* and the questions below, remember to watch the process of what you do to avoid things, not judge it. When we judge ourselves and our actions too quickly, we miss the importance of the process itself. For now, watch how much of your orientation is toward avoiding what you don't want and notice what falls into your avoidance category (what you dislike will be different than someone else). Notice what you do to avoid. Feel and sense in your body and nervous system what is happening as you push something away. Remember, we are trying to know ourselves, not fix ourselves.

Reflection: Make a list of things you avoid (people, food, places, music, colors, smells, etc.). Now reflect on how this list came to be.

Reflection: Notice how much of your day, attention, and energy goes into avoidance. How might this avoidance be an accommodation of your weaknesses / your conditioning?

Reflection: Notice where and how you lay your own anger or selfishness on someone or something else. Notice if it's because you didn't get what you wanted.

Reflection: Avoid the tendency to use adjectives and adverbs. Practice naming things without using descriptive words. Can you just let things be?

Abhinivesha ~ FEARING DEATH / LOSS / CHANGE

Studies show that as we age, the majority of us have less subjects to talk about. The wonder and enthusiasm we had as children for just about everything has turned into a litany of complaints about our aches and pains and comments on the weather. This is the work of *abhinivesha*, the fifth *klesha*.

Not knowing who we really are (*avidya*), mistaking ourselves for who we think we are (*asmita*), clinging to what we think will make us happy (*raga*), and resisting what makes us unhappy (*dvesha*) has brought us to the state of *abhinivesha*—afraid of just about everything.

Here, we find ourselves afraid of just about everything. We are afraid of dying, afraid of not having what we want, afraid of losing what we have, afraid of getting what we don't want, afraid of change. We cling, at times desperately, to the life we know.

I am reminded of a song written in the 1960's by Micky Newbury called "Just Dropped In (To See What Condition My Condition Is In)." Although written to warn of the dangers of LSD, the lyrics keep playing in my head as I write this chapter. Perhaps it's because if we do "drop in to see what condition our condition is in," we might be surprised to discover how robotic and fearful we have become.

We continue to demand that life meet us on our own terms. We fail to notice some of the odd behavior, poor choices, and compensations that have become part of our lives. We follow a familiar downward spiral into rigidity, fear, and anxiety. We remain unwilling to give more than lip service to the unavoidable reality that someday we will die.

It is interesting to me how significantly the book, *Being Mortal: Medicine and What Matters in the End*, by Atul Gawande has impacted so many peoples' hearts and minds. The book offers an honest assessment of health care, autonomy, aging, choices, and real conversations about our wishes with those we love. I think many have found comfort in the sincere conversation about death rather than the avoidance that pervades our Western culture.

To revisit our snow analogy, if we forget that everything is snow and instead cling to the forms made of snow, we live in constant fear of losing these forms. We fear the warming temperatures and do everything in our power to protect ourselves and the things we love from melting. The brilliancy of our minds and our creative ability, instead of being focused on art, service, and discovering our full potential, gets focused on protecting what we have.

Not only does *abhinivesha* seep into every aspect of our life; it has its own sustaining power continually enforcing its rigidity. In the process, it creates suffering for others, as well as the earth herself. It produces both local and worldwide challenges, that, when we are prisoners of this *klesha*, we are simply not qualified to meet.

My spouse and I were compelled to watch the 10-part documentary on the Vietnam War by Ken Burns and Lynn Novick. This is the era we grew up in. These were our friends that were killed. This is the war that shaped our thinking.

At that time, there was a contagious fear of communism and a prevailing belief in the so-called domino effect. It was understood that if one country fell under communist rule, so would the next and the next, like a well-placed set of dominoes, that have no choice but to fall as the next falling domino in turn knocks it over.

Not only did this belief prevail, but we, as citizens of the United States, were high on ourselves. We could do no wrong. We were the great leader of democracy and the savior of the world. Our fear, our arrogance, and our savior-complex led to a kind of tyrannical thinking. We assumed we were right, so we didn't question.

Our political leaders (spanning five presidents) saw we were losing the war. Instead of admitting this, they continued to add more troops, continued to prop up an unpopular and unjust government in South Vietnam, and increased the bombing in North Vietnam. Policy had been enforced to the point of rigidity, leading to more death, destruction, and suffering.

In *The Butter Battle Book* by Dr. Seuss, a wall separates the Yooks who live on one side, from the Zooks who live on the other. The Yooks and the Zooks have become enemies over how bread and butter should be eaten. The Yooks eat their bread butter side up and the Zooks eat theirs butter side down. An escalating war ensues between the two sides as new weapons of destruction are manufactured. Eventually both sides have the capability to blow the other side up.

The story illustrates how the rigidity of *abhinivesha* can affect behavior. We can see the absurdity of escalating a war over the "correct" way to eat bread and butter. Yet, caught in our own rigidity, there is a blindness to what we can see and how we are prone to see it. Cognitive ability and perception get channeled into a familiar groove. We can't think outside the box. We don't even know we are in a box! We've locked life into a routine of familiarity. Stuck in *abhinivesha*, the always new, vastly unlimited, creative potential in each of us gets stymied.

As I wrote this chapter, I had been called up for two weeks of jury duty. As some of you may know, the courthouse records a message that will play after 5pm, letting those of us on call know if we are required to show up at court the following day. For two nights I made my evening call, but the phone continued to ring on the other end. I continued to call the courthouse number several times, but the result was the same; there was no recorded message.

My mind was full of complaints, all directed at the incompetency of the courthouse. My body became agitated by my growing frustration. On the third night, after getting the same results, I indignantly showed my spouse the instruction letter I had received in the mail. He quickly pointed out that I had been calling the wrong number.

Of course, I felt quite stupid, but that is the point. So often in our own limited place of understanding, we blame the other while we self-righteously stand in our own ignorance. I probably would have faced some contempt of court charges; fortunately, I had not been requested to show up. But still, damage had been done in the form of the internal chaos this whole ordeal caused to my mind and also to my spouse. As I had spiraled deeper into entanglement, the ability to recognize the possibility that I was in the wrong became impossible.

My Uncle Bill died at the age of 92 in physical pain, but mentally alert, and with spiritual security. He was considered by many to be a giant of a human being. Shortly before he died, circumstances brought me to his bedside where I took the opportunity to seek the wisdom carried by one who had lived long and learned well along the way.

Sitting by my Uncle Bill, I asked him, "What do you regret the most in your life?" His eyes turned reflectively inward as he answered, "I grew up in a community of immigrants from four different countries, all speaking their native language and living out their unique customs. In all the opportunity there was for me to play with children who had come from a country different than my own, I chose instead to play with the German boys because that was what I knew. I could have learned new words, played new games, tasted different food, and made new friends, but I chose to stay 'with my own kind.' I regret to this day that I missed out on so much."

It's hard to convey the tangible heaviness in Uncle Bill's voice as he spoke; it's also hard to convey my own surprise that in 92 years of living this would be his biggest regret. But I witnessed the cost to my uncle, and I am witnessing it today in a world that seems bent on protecting what is familiar and feeling threatened by what is different.

Without awareness of the *kleshas*, it is difficult to see what sits beyond our limited world of perceived reality. Even when we are aware, we don't seem to know how to free ourselves from these deep-seated messages. Since all we know is what we know, we often try to do more of the same thing to get a different result, but nothing really changes.

My spouse and I were feeling stressed because we were far behind with our work. We came up with a brilliant plan, or so we thought. We decided to support each other to get up at 3:00 am every morning for two weeks, thinking we could get caught up and then life would be so much easier. Suffice it to say that after two weeks of 3:00 am coffee and catch up, all we had to show for it was exhaustion and a gloomy sense of defeat.

In this place of wanting things to be different, we often end up exhausting ourselves as we keep doing more of the same while hoping for a different outcome. We see this action in politics, business, and various organizations, as well as in our own lives. We are unable to examine the belief that is driving us and the fear that keeps us from doing what really needs to be done, and so we keep throwing more of the same at it hoping for a different outcome. A different outcome never comes.

For my spouse and I, we had not yet been able to entertain the concept that perhaps we had agreed to do more than was humanly possible, and what we needed was to let go of some of our commitments. The cost to us was a stressful and unbalanced life.

In some areas of our lives, we have followed the formula for success and it has worked. We have attained the image of success; we are now secure. We have arrived at the completion of our goal. Now we become the protectors of the status quo. We become the storytellers of success and proof of the "correct" way to be. Although our life appears to be working, the limits of our success show up as arrogant entitlement, a strange loneliness, and always the undercurrent of anxiety over our imminent death.

> Unaware of these deep-seated beliefs in control of our lives, we pass these limits, along with any trauma they have caused, on to our children and students. This is the human condition.

Unaware of these deep-seated beliefs in control of our lives, we pass these limits, along with any trauma they have caused, on to our children and students. This is the human condition. This is the natural process of lived humanity unless something breaks in to shift our thinking, to make us aware of our own ignorance and the way we cling to this ignorance. Somehow, over time, we become comfortable in our habits.

For some, habits have led to a certain success and enjoyment of life; for others, habits have led to a kind of miserable comfortableness. Either way, our habits eventually produce a sense of security that imprisons us to varying degrees. We can feel the discontentment, the pull to adventure, the desire to burst ourselves on the world and see what can happen. Yet we may easily settle for the comfort and safety of the habitual life that has, in part, been created for us.

Although *abhinivesha* is often a gloomy scenario, we do have choices. Even if our beliefs and conditioning do not go away, we can examine and reflect on them. Even if our limitations do not go away, we can be more expansive and open within these limitations. Even if our preferences do not go away, we can learn a different standard from which to judge our happiness.

I close this chapter with a reflection by Jett Sophia. I have carried this with me for several years. I have found it a helpful way to reflect on beliefs and find some wiggle room within clinging to life as I know it.

> I stalk beliefs. I lurk around the corners of my mind, listening to what I think and to what I say, ready to pounce when a belief appears. When I

catch one, I investigate it. Becoming as open and undefended as I can, I try the belief on. What is its purpose? How does it feel in/on my body?

By and large, their purpose, it seems to me, is to make me feel safe, to make me feel less bewildered about the situations of life. But when I feel my way into beliefs, they almost always feel something like being encased in cotton batting, sticky cotton batting. They inhibit my breath, they cling to my skin, they make me feel energetically murky.

Safety takes up space that could be occupied by glory, by wonder, by awe, by curiosity. Glory, wonder, awe, joy, endless possibility — they feel spacious, airy, bright. There is no contest — they feel way better than sticky cotton batting.

So I stalk beliefs. I lurk and I pounce. And when I catch one, I celebrate. Because then I have a choice to either keep it or release it.

~ Jett Sophia, *Signal Fire* © 2012 & 2022

Questions for Reflection

As you reflect on *abhinivesha* and the questions below, remember that by this point the *kleshas* have taken on a self-perpetuating quality; the content of the *kleshas* determines what we think about, the choices we make, and the actions we take.

Reflection: Where are you throwing energy at parts of your life that aren't working? What might change if you examined your conditioning rather than trying to make your conditioning work?

Reflection: In what ways or in what areas of your life do you experience rigidity? In what ways does this feel like a loss of vitality or hopelessness or just plain being stuck? Can you trace this sense of rigidity back through the tightening grip of *abhinivesha*? (Note the difference between healthy routines that provide a framework for growth and the experience of being stuck.)

Reflection: Name a couple of fears. In what ways can you trace these fears back to *abhinivesha*? What do these fears keep you from doing that you really want to do?
Name a couple of regrets. In what ways can you trace these regrets back to *abhinivesha*? How do these regrets clog your mind and keep you ruminating about the past?

Reflection: In the words of Jett Sophia, stalk a belief or two and pounce on them. Then investigate them. What do they feel like?

Considerations

Writing about the *kleshas* has been an interesting process for me. Much like my experience with the *yamas* and *niyamas*, I thought I had a good grasp of these concepts (I taught them for years), and I thought I was pretty much free of them. Ha! What arrogance. Having written these chapters, I am more than humbled to see my utter captivity in them. And without doubt, I have just scratched the surface.

It has been a hard process, not the writing itself so much as the "seeing" how these *kleshas* insert themselves into every corner of my existence. At times it has felt "dark," but at the same time strangely freeing. I had to ask, "Is orienting my life around my personal pleasure all my life is about? Are the knee-jerk emotional reactions to things that don't go my way worth the strain on my body? How much have I been missing out on by insisting life fit my agenda?"

I share this process now because the growing ability to see my captivity feels like bursts of pure grace. And maybe that is what Patanjali was hoping for. Perhaps knowledge of the *kleshas* is a life-saving compassion that fuels awareness and discipline. Krishna says to Arjuna in chapter six of the Bhagavad Gita that the real meaning of yoga is deliverance from contact with pain and suffering.

Patanjali is clear, it is our entanglement in the *kleshas* that gives rise to suffering and misery by creating a whole misguided narrative of reality. Patanjali is also clear, there is a way out. We are not here to suffer and to cause suffering to others. We are not here to be protective, afraid, needy, defensive, conflicted, and judgmental. There is an entirely different reality than the one the *kleshas* present, and it is always new and expansive, always now.

What is the practice that can help us see what we don't know how to see? Sometimes it is great loss or turbulent social times that stir us out of our slumber and turn us towards deep reflection. Kate Bowler is one such example. She did everything "right" according to the narrative

> What is the practice that can help us see what we don't know how to see?

that defined her reality. A professor at Duke University, happily enjoying her marriage and life with her newborn son, she believed that blessings in life meant God approved of you; hardships were a sign of God's disapproval. At 35 she was diagnosed with stage 4 cancer, and suddenly the narrative she had lived by made no sense. She writes about her process of questioning her beliefs in the New York Times best seller, *Everything Happens for a Reason: And Other Lies I've Loved.*

This is only one example of the myriad of personal and communal events that come unsolicited and unwelcome and land on the doorstep of our perceived reality. When they do come, we have the opportunity to look at our beliefs and question their validity….or to complain, blame, and stay rigid in our thinking.

For many of us, it is a chosen spiritual discipline that puts us on a path of reflective introspection and breaks us open to new possibilities. All too often a spiritual discipline is thought to be a place of comfort and serenity. And this is true; it is a refuge.

Often, a spiritual discipline is thought to be a place of comfort and serenity. And this is true; it is a refuge. But the purpose of a spiritual path is also to turn our world upside down and inside out.

But the purpose of a spiritual path is also to turn our world upside down and inside out. The purpose is to help us see what we don't know how to see and to know what we don't know how to know. It is to help us open our eyes to complexity, paradox, mystery, and the vulnerability of not knowing. It is to help us meet life joyfully and skillfully on its own terms, rather than demanding life subject itself to our personal whims. It is to deliver us from fear and the suffering caused by our own misperceptions.

Yet our total entanglement into seeking pleasure and avoiding pain can sneak its way into our spiritual practice. For instance, we might ask ourselves, am I doing my spiritual practice to be good or to be real? Our co-dependency and addictions stem from our desire to feel good and not to feel bad. This can apply to our gratitude practices and positive affirmations as well as our habit of reaching for a glass of wine or updates on social media.

At the core of our suffering, Patanjali tells us, is our need to have things on our own terms and that means keeping the self-defined good stuff coming and keeping the self-defined bad stuff at bay. This pattern becomes self-perpetuating. If we don't recognize this pattern, our spiritual practice easily takes on the quality of seeking what feels good and avoiding what feels bad, with the goal of eventually attaining a self-defined paradise. In the process, we can continue to judge others rather than face the tendencies that live within us.

The very practice that is designed to take us out of our entanglement in the *kleshas* may end up being a practice that keeps us in our entanglement. I raise this point now, so that as we move into looking at Patanjali's plan for becoming free of the *kleshas* we might look at the practice through different eyes. If we don't understand that we bring our pleasure seeking/pain avoiding selves with us into our yoga practice, our practice may perpetuate this pattern, not free us from it.

We need a practice that will take us out of our rigidity, not satisfy it. We need a practice that will teach us a different way of finding nurturance than getting our likes satisfied and keeping our dislikes at bay. We need a practice that will rock our sense of identity, not agree with it. We need a practice that will show us our ignorance, not reinforce it. We need a practice that will expose our narrative, not fit nicely within it.

I am reminded of the movie *The Matrix* where Neo is given the choice of taking the red pill or the blue pill. Swallowing one pill insures he can stay in the world as he knows it. Swallowing the other pill will unplug him from the narrative he is familiar with and set him on a path that shows him a very different reality. Once we are awake to the *kleshas*, we have a similar choice. We can willingly remain their captive, or we can begin a path of healing and transformation that will open up a new reality to us, and in the process free us from our captivity and suffering.

Patanjali, in the Yoga Sutra, defines such a path for us; it is a path of practice coupled with nonattachment that will take us from being bound/entangled in the *kleshas* to freedom from the *kleshas*. In this process, it is critical to understand the importance of the mind, because the mind is the platform where it all happens.

Mind

THE PLATFORM

*So if you, like me, ever wondered
what the mind has to do with things,
the answer is, well, everything.*

I was an avid student and practitioner of yoga for years before I knew that yoga had anything to do with the mind. How this important fact escaped my understanding is beyond me. One day something changed as I read some words by Georg Feuerstein. He spoke to the fact that everything happens in the mind; it is in the mind that we are captured by the *kleshas* or freed from them.

To say that I immediately understood the importance of his words would be inaccurate. The idea that the mind was where everything happened puzzled me. I pondered this idea until one day I sat down and made a simple sketch to help bring clarity to the idea that the mind can orient toward bondage, or the mind can orient toward freedom.

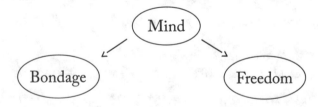

Once I had sketched this diagram, it became the centerpiece of my curiosity. Up until that time, I never thought much about my mind except to ask a lot of it, and even that was not a conscious ask. The main relationship I had with my mind was to get agitated when I couldn't remember someone's name. Now, the mind as the place where my bondage and freedom happened was all I could think about.

At the time, I was co-owner of a yoga studio, a perfect place to explore learning with like-minded people. Gathering what little knowledge I had and could find, I offered the first 6-month Mind Study in 2006. I chose *Conquest of Mind* by Eknath Easwaran as our text, created weekly experiments (like doing things we wouldn't normally do), and shaped our monthly inquiry around pertinent quotes that gave us insights into the mind.

The simple act of inquiring about the mind instead of taking it for granted was new for all of us and valuable in itself. It was a study that we continued year after year with great interest.

So if you, like me, ever wondered what the mind has to do with things, the answer is, well, everything.

The Role of the Mind

Often when teaching class, I have asked participants what their definition of yoga is. What follows are many beautiful responses like health, freedom, contentment, etc., all of which are true. Never have I heard someone mention the mind in their definition. Yet in chapter 1, verse 2 of the Yoga Sutra, Patanjali defines yoga as "Complete mastery over the roaming tendencies of the mind" (Tigunait, p. 5). Apparently, yoga has everything to do with the mind.

We spent a whole section discussing the *kleshas*, and now we are talking about the mind and the roaming tendencies. Let's see if we can start putting this together. Have you ever sat down to balance your finances and been unable to focus on the task at hand? Or sat down to meditate, determined to stay focused on your breath only to find it didn't take long before your mind had "roamed" far from your breath to something entirely different? Even though you intended to stay focused, your mind, it seemed, had a very different idea.

What is the power that pulls the mind to these places? You guessed it, the *kleshas*. Ah, now it is starting to make sense. The Sanskrit word for roaming tendencies is *vrittis*, literally meaning "to whirl" or "to spin." Our minds, which have an inherent nature of tranquility, have become enamored with the *kleshas*. This process is somewhat like the flowing water of a creek. The water's natural state is to flow peacefully, yet in places where there are clusters of rocks, the water whirls and sometimes foams from the obstacles created by the rocks.

Our limited concept of reality (*avidya*), our limited understanding of ourselves (*asmita*), our likes (*raga*), our dislikes (*dvesha*), and the rigidity that ensues from our fear of loss / death / change (*abhinivesha*) live in the mind. This is what the mind knows, and it imposes its own limited viewpoint onto the larger world. It sees its own conditioning and beliefs reflected everywhere and calls it reality.

Though invisible, the *kleshas* are a potent blockage to the peaceful flowing energy of the mind. Like water whirling around a rock, the mind roams around the *kleshas*, disrupting tranquility. The continuous roaming of the mind around the *kleshas* creates patterns of thoughts and actions that solidify habits (*samskaras*) and deep subtle impressions (*vasanas*), taking us deeper into bondage. The result of these habits and subtle impressions is the creation of *karma* that in turn creates lifetime after lifetime of births and deaths (*samsara*) lived out in the same *klesha*-created pattern of afflictions. (Note: Although reincarnation exists in yoga philosophy, it is not necessary to believe in reincarnation to benefit from yogic insights into the *kleshas* and the disturbances of the mind.)

Key to all of this is recognizing that the intrinsic, natural state of the mind is clear and peaceful. No roaming tendencies, just a pure lens or mirror that sees without distortion. The *kleshas* may be present, but the mind isn't reacting to them. This is an important point as yoga is not a war on the *kleshas* but the ability to not be disturbed or misled by them.

For me it is difficult to comprehend that the natural state of the mind is tranquil; that is not my usual experience.

But there is something important here. If the innate state of the mind is tranquil, then the experience of disturbance, scatteredness, and dullness is not natural; it has been learned. And thus, it can be unlearned. This is good news.

> If the innate state of the mind is tranquil, then the experience of disturbance, scatteredness, and dullness is not natural; it has been learned. And thus, it can be unlearned. This is good news.

The other good news is, according to Patanjali, we are not everything that is happening to us; we are not even what we are thinking. The roaming of our minds causes us to identify with the contents of our minds, but it is a false identification. To know who we really are requires a stilling of the mind's proclivity to wander in order to reveal what is hidden beneath the wandering.

Patanjali explains this process succinctly in the first four verses of the Yoga Sutra:

> YS 1.1. "Now begins the instruction on the practice of Yoga."
> YS 1.2. "Complete mastery over the roaming tendencies of the mind is Yoga."
> YS 1.3. "Then the Seer becomes established in its essential nature."
> YS 1.4. "Elsewhere [the Seer] conforms to the roaming tendencies of the mind" (Tigunait, pgs. 1, 4, 10, 14).

Putting down our scholarly hat, we could paraphrase Patanjali something like this: (1) Here is what yoga is. (2) Yoga is mastering the mind's habit to roam. (3) If you master the mind's roaming, the mind will be in its innate pure nature and you will rest in your true essence. (4) If you don't master the mind's roaming, you will continue to suffer afflictions.

What Patanjali is teaching is similar to Buddha's first words as he experienced his awakening after sitting for days under the bodhi tree. Buddha noted that there is suffering, and yet there doesn't have to be suffering. Then he said that there is a way out of suffering and he taught the path to freedom.

Several years ago I was invited to teach at a studio in Pennsylvania. The studio owner graciously invited me to stay in her home where she resided with her partner, five dogs, and one cat. It was lively, to say the least. While in their home, I noticed a large bookcase filled with several books about dogs. One in particular which caught my eye was called *How to Raise a Puppy You Can Live With*. "Oh," I thought to myself, "This is what yoga is; it is how to raise a mind you can live with."

The mind is the key to freedom, but what is the mind, and how is it different than the brain?

The Brain / Mind Distinction

The words brain and mind get used in interesting ways. I remember my dad telling me to "use my brain" when I had done something foolish. He also referred to people he considered intelligent as having a lot of "brain power."

The word mind is used in phrases such as "I have a good mind to…," "I'll keep that in mind," "You were on my mind," "I'm going to give them a piece of my mind," "She's out of her mind," "I wish they would make up their mind," and "She displays a great presence of mind."

To confuse things more, the words brain and mind often get used interchangeably as if they are the same. But are they? Turning to western science, which focuses on the brain, and yogic science, which focuses on the mind, we can begin to discern the difference.

In 1989, George H.W. Bush signed a presidential declaration designating the 1990's as the "Decade of the Brain," a focus that gave neuroscience a prominent standing. During that time, technological advances in high-powered microscopes, imaging tools, and computer simulation allowed scientists to see the brain in ways never before possible.

Much was learned about the brain, but the distinction between brain and mind remained hazy. Scientists agreed that the brain was a mechanism that energy and information flow through. They could literally watch this process happen in the brain. The mind, however, remained somewhat nebulous and hard to define. What was understood was that how the energy and information get modulated belonged to the domain of mind.

In other words, we know a lot about the brain and how it sends information via chemical hormones and electrical currents. But how this objective information gets translated into a personal, subjective experience (the work of the mind), remains a mystery.

Think about this for a minute. There is something about each one of us that is able to make an electrical/chemical impulse into a real, lived, felt experience. Furthermore, how we interpret this electrical/chemical information determines whether we add to our own (and others') suffering or to our own (and others') wellbeing.

The brain is tangible; we can hold it in our hands, dissect it, and perform surgery on it. With the use of powerful microscopes, we can watch the input and output of sensory exchange. We can see where in the brain the centers of speech, vision, fear, emotions, instincts, logical thinking, and memory are located.

The mind, however, is not tangible. We can't see it or hold it in our hands. We can't dissect it, perform surgery on it, or watch its process. We can't physically see the beliefs, conditioning, trauma, wounds, clinging and resisting that are integral to the process of the mind's interpretation. On Election Day, I vote for one party; my neighbor votes for another. Walking with my spouse, I see trees and clouds; he sees cars and people. The same chemical/electrical process is happening in the brain, but the personal interpretation creates different responses.

We owe much to leading neuroscientists and the knowledge they have gained from their extensive research. Words like default mode network (the auto-pilot mode the brain resorts to when not cognitively focused), negativity bias (the tendency to pay attention to what is considered undesirable), neuroception (the ability to gauge the perception of safety), and neuroplasticity (the ability of the brain to change depending on how it is used) are now part of the common vernacular. Phrases like "neurons that fire together, wire together" are a reminder that what we keep doing, is what we keep doing. Numerous children's books are now available teaching children the value of having a flexible brain.

Research validates the positive or negative impact chemicals released from our brain have on our health. A fear-based, anxious reaction to an experience creates a toxic environment for our cells. A joyful, trustful reaction creates an environment in which our cells can thrive. These chemicals influence gene expression and epigenetics, affect the length of our telomeres, alter our immune system, and change the microbiome in our gut depending on the environment that is produced based on our personal reaction to an experience.

Not only has neuroscience advanced our knowledge of the brain, it has also provided insights into the mind, and validation for what yogis experienced thousands of years ago.

Reflection: Setting aside all knowledge you have about the brain and the mind, answer the following questions from a place of your experiential knowledge. What do you know about the brain/mind because you have one, not because you have read about them? What do you personally mean when you use the word brain or mind? How do you commonly use these words? What is your personal experience of having a brain? A mind?

Reflection: Sit with these words from Dr. David Frawley: "We are so caught up in the mind's activities that we do not take the time to discover what the mind itself really is" (Frawley, p. 43).

Yogic Understanding of the Mind

The Sanskrit word for mind is *antahkarana* meaning "the inner instrument." Mind is the tool, or instrument, through which consciousness looks at the world and sees itself (somewhat like we look in a mirror and see ourselves). In the same manner that brain is a tool of mind, mind is a tool of consciousness. And consciousness is pure awareness with the power to be aware of itself. Yogis agree that the mind is a mystery, but where western science has much to contribute to the brain, yogic science contributes understanding to the mystery of the mind.

> Mind is the tool, or instrument, through which consciousness looks at the world and sees itself. In the same manner that brain is a tool of mind, mind is a tool of consciousness. And consciousness is pure awareness with the power to be aware of itself.

It is the mind that shapes our reality by giving us a sense of time, space, and cause & effect. In other words, we experience things in a linear fashion, happening within space, and getting a result (effect) from the action we took (cause). These three ways of experiencing the happenings of our life shape our reality in ways we take for granted.

Although it is easy to think of the mind as a tangible "thing," it is made of the subtlest form of energy. As energy, its nature is to move and to change. Think how quickly our experience of peacefulness (a tranquil state known as *sattva*) can change into an agitated, distracted experience (an active state known as *rajas*) or a dull, stale experience (a stupefied state known as *tamas*). This change can be caused by passive reactions to the *klesha* experience or it can be intentionally directed. In our practice, it is important to remember that the mind is moving energy, and we have the power to direct that energy. This is why the mind can change its orientation from roaming to stillness.

Where is the mind located? In the brain? In the body? Outside the body?

We also might consider where the mind is located and discover that it is difficult to pinpoint its whereabouts. Does it exist in the brain? In the body? Outside the body? Yogic thinking tells us that all of the body is in the mind, but not all of the mind is in the body. In other words, the mind includes the body but is more than the body. In like manner, all of the mind is in consciousness, but not all of consciousness is in the mind.

Where the mind resides is important. In the west we tend to think of ourselves as a brain in our head that drags the body along. But if the *kleshas* live in our mind, and all of the body is in the mind, then the *kleshas* live in our nervous system and our tissues, as well as the energy field around us.

The mind is a storehouse of past impressions and information. Everything we have been taught, experienced, and dreamed is cataloged and kept somewhere in the recesses of our mind. Some of it is easily accessible, and some gets forgotten, or so it seems. Some events get lumped together and the details get hazy and somewhat inaccurate. Some experiences remain in the conscious memory while others get relegated to the depths of the unconscious.

In past travels to visit parents, I used to drive by an Amazon warehouse. The sheer size of the building was staggering. I knew that inside there were rows of shelving with stacked products many layers high. The inventory was of monumental numbers, and the categorizing system impressive. Our minds are much like this warehouse, storing all the pieces of our individual lives.

Ideally, all this stored information serves to help navigate our lives well, but bondage to the *kleshas* creates a different scenario. When we cling to beliefs, ideas, people, and objects we are unwilling to let go of (*raga*), it's as if we have installed bright lights, security cameras, tall fences, and guards to vigilantly protect these things. In a strange way, we do the same thing to what we avoid and resist (*dvesha*); we diligently guard them to keep them at bay. Instead of a peaceful working environment, our minds are constantly taxed to keep and increase the things we value, as well as to keep the things we find distasteful away.

All of the above happens when we have unfinished business, undigested experience, trauma (our own plus what we've inherited generationally), wounds, scars…whatever we call it, these are the places that trip up the mind's peaceful flow of energy. They are much like undigested food in the body that sticks around long after it should have been either assimilated or eliminated. Unless something is done to process these particles, disease and loss of vitality follow.

The people, things, and beliefs we won't let go of, the people, things, and beliefs we won't let near us, and the experiences we've not fully integrated into or eliminated from our lives are the things that the mind roams around. Rather than experiencing a peaceful flowing mind, we experience a mind that is hyper-vigilant, scattered, and mostly exhausted. Rather than experience each moment, we are busy telling ourselves about the moment.

> Rather than experience each moment, we are busy telling ourselves about the moment.

This is the mind most of us are familiar with, the mind that has an opinion about, well, just about everything. It likes to compare, judge, criticize, praise, blame, analyze, figure out, etc. It puts adjectives and adverbs on everything based on the content of its conditioning. The mind's essence is pure, but a mind captivated by the *kleshas* is a mind that roams.

Reflection: What is it like to think of your mind as subtle energy that is always moving? Does this change the usual way you think of your mind? In what way?

Reflection: What is it like to think of your mind as including, but more than, your body? Does anything change when you have a sense of yourself in this proportion?

The Functions of the Mind

When Patanjali discusses the mind, he is focused on the
roaming tendencies (*vrittis*) that disturb the innate quality
of the mind. He categorizes the *vrittis* into five types: right
knowledge, wrong knowledge, imagination, memory, and
sleep (Yoga Sutra 1:6-11). He adds that these five categories
can be *klish* or *aklish*, painful or nonpainful (Yoga Sutra
1:5). Even though all roaming tendencies interfere with the
inherent quality of the mind, it is worth contemplating the
effect of painful thoughts and nonpainful thoughts.

Vedanta Yoga, one of the six systems of Vedic philosophy,
explores the mind by looking at the four functions or
processes that the mind coordinates. The functions are
known as *manas* (the importer and exporter of sensory
data), *ahamkara* (the ego), *buddhi* (the ability to witness and
discern), and *chitta* (the individual storehouse of personal
experience). (Note: While Patanjali uses the word *chitta* to
refer to the mind itself, Vedanta uses the word *chitta* to refer
to the storehouse or mind field of personal experience.)

Understanding these functions and their interconnection
sheds light on how we find ourselves believing what
our roaming, thinking mind tells us even as we long for
something different. We have already explored the personal
storehouse of memory and experience that each of us carry.
Now we turn to the remaining three functions.

Ahamkara ~ THE EGO

Have you ever wondered what makes each of us feel like us? Or what creates an "us" and "them"? Or why some things feel personal to us and not to others? For the yogis, this reality is created by a process of the mind called *ahamkara*, a Sanskrit word meaning "I-maker."

Ahamkara is the function of the mind we refer to as ego. Ego creates the experience of "I" by drawing a boundary around itself. It creates the feeling "this is me" and "this isn't me." If you are familiar with Saturday Night Live, you might remember Chevy Chase saying, "I'm Chevy Chase, and you're not!" The audience responded with laughter, but in truth, when Chevy said those words, he nailed *ahamkara*.

> The way we know ourselves as a separate entity is created by an invisible boundary we draw around ourselves and then experience the separateness as real.

If we stop to take this in, the process seems rather fascinating. The way we know ourselves as a separate entity is created by an invisible boundary we draw around ourselves and then experience the separateness as real. *Ahamkara* is for all practical purposes the same as *asmita*. The subtle difference is that *ahamkara* creates the boundary (I am a separate entity), and *asmita* labels what is inside the boundary (I am successful, I am a mother). We think of ourselves as the contents inside the boundary.

Experiencing ourselves as existing within a boundary makes everything feel personal. We each experience ourselves as subject and everything else as object. (Our language uses first person and third person to denote this experience.) When everything feels personal, it raises the stakes of the experience. Rather than say "a belief," we say "my belief." The possessiveness causes a deeper investment and entanglement. We can feel threatened and volatile when someone disagrees with us because the belief feels like part of us.

> To learn to create a peaceful inner world is the crux of the teachings of all great spiritual traditions.

Experiencing ourselves as a separate entity also necessitates ego's need to constantly do something. It needs to figure something out, fix something, plan something, or create conflict with others. All these enliven the sense of separateness and give the ego a sense of misplaced power. We assume we are the doer; we are the thinker; we are the knower.

The boundary made by ego creates an experience of two worlds, one we experience as "in here" and one we experience as "out there." The inner world is unique to each of us; we are each the only one inside ourselves. It is here, Patanjali tells us, that both our bondage and our liberation happen. To learn to create a peaceful inner world is the crux of the teachings of all great spiritual traditions. To understand that this is the place we have complete jurisdiction, is to awaken to spiritual discipline.

But it is the "out there," the place we interact with people and objects we don't identify as ourselves, that pulls our attention away from the "in here." Because we know ourselves in relation to our environment, we are compelled to pay attention to the environment for both safety and acceptance. This constant pull to the outer world keeps us cautious and vigilant, as we cling to and resist people and events in a misguided attempt to feel safe, accepted, and fulfilled. With our focus "out there," the senses become a powerful force in determining our lives.

To understand how this interaction between the inner world and the outer world happens, we turn our attention to the senses and a function of the mind called *manas*.

Reflection: Explore the function known as *ahamkara*, or ego. Notice how some things feel personal and others don't. Explore this experience in terms of what you consider to be "you" and "not you." What does this have to do with empathy and caring what happens to others?

Reflection: Practice replacing "my" with "a" this week. In other words instead of saying "my" belief, say "a" belief. Replace "my" book with "a" book, etc. Does this shift in possessive language make a difference in how you see things? What do you notice?

Manas ~ IMPORTER & EXPORTER OF SENSORY DATA

Unlike the inner world, which is a personal, subjective world, the outer world is a shared, objective one. We experience earth, rain, sky, sun, trees, animals, and other humans. We share (or argue over) beliefs, rules and regulations, and codes of conduct for sharing this space.

At the boundary between these two worlds is our skin and sense organs; it is the senses that provide the medium of exchange that allows for our relational experience with the outer world. How does this exchange happen? Through *manas*, a function of the mind whose job is to import and export sensory data. *Manas* is sometimes fondly referred to as the "monkey mind" because of its constant chatter, a term that captures the busyness of our minds as they are almost constantly bombarded by sensory stimulation.

Relationships happen through a give and take exchange. There is some form of information coming in and some form of information that responds. There are five senses that import information to us in the form of smelling, tasting, seeing, touching, and hearing. These are called the senses of cognition; it is the manner in which we take in the people and objects we experience as outside of us, or the outer world.

But we have five more senses that allow us to act on the world. Information comes in through the five senses of cognition, and we have the choice of if and how we will respond through five additional senses called the senses of action. These are elimination, reproduction/creation,

locomotion, grasping, and speaking. All of this allows
for the experience of relationship and exchange with our
environment, a constant input and output of sensory
information and choice.

Exchange with the Outer World Happens Through:	
Senses of Cognition (Input)	Senses of Action (Output)
Hear	Speak
Touch	Grasp
See	Move
Taste	Reproduce/Create
Smell	Eliminate

In the nervous system, which directs all the body's activities,
this interaction happens through the afferent and efferent
neurons. Afferent neurons, referred to as the sensory neurons,
carry information from the sensory organs to the central
nervous system while efferent neurons, referred to as the
motor neurons, carry nerve impulses from the central nervous
system to the muscles.

It is a simple in and out process that allows exchange and
thus experience to happen. It can be a profound, enriching
process that brings enjoyment and pleasure to all participants,
unless the mind is expecting lasting happiness from the
sensory exchange. Trying to sustain the pleasure one scoop
of ice cream gives leads to overindulgence and a body in
complaint. Trying to sustain the fullness of an intimate
moment with a friend or life partner sets them up for certain

failure. Trying to sustain the pleasure of a newly purchased item soon disappoints and leads to more purchases.

The uncontrollable and constant seeking of happiness through sensory pleasure is likened to a chariot drawn by ten horses (Katha Upanishad). In this image, the chariot represents the physical body and the ten horses represent the ten senses. When the horses are allowed to go wherever they want, the chariot gets beaten up. In like manner, when our senses are allowed to indulge, they can lead us to overeat, overbuy, or spend too much time in the metaverse. The result is a body that, like the chariot, gets beaten up.

When we seek to satisfy our cravings without asking what it is we are really craving, when we believe our thoughts without examining them, when we allow the outer world to draw us away from our inner stability, we live in bondage.

There is no denying it, sensory pleasures are, well, pleasurable, and the outer world is compelling. But as long as the senses are left to indulge as they please and to be constantly allured by the next inviting thing, we suffer. When we take without giving back, when we take more than our share, when we succeed on the backs of others, we are violating the law of reciprocity. Living without respect and restraint insures physical, mental, and emotional pain for ourselves and others.

When we seek to satisfy our cravings without asking what it is we are really craving, when we believe our thoughts without examining them, when we allow the outer world to draw us away from our inner stability, we live in bondage. It is as if we have set the cruise control in our car and are driving steadily along the highway named *abhinivesha* (fear of loss / fear of change / fear of death).

Thankfully there is a function of the mind that allows us to see when we are going in the wrong direction. It is a function that allows us to see what it is we are really craving. It is a function that allows us to examine our thoughts and to stay inside ourselves. This function is called *buddhi*, or "higher mind," and it provides us the opportunity to break out of bondage.

Reflection: Explore the function known as *manas*, the importer and exporter of sensory data. Notice the exchange between "you" and the "outer world." In what ways do you experience the power of sensory stimulation? How do you take in and act on this information in terms of your particular need for safety, resources, and approval? Notice how alluring this whole process is.

Reflection: Notice the difference between enjoying the senses and being a prisoner to them.

Buddhi ~ THE HIGHER MIND

The word *buddhi* means "awake." Think of Buddha, who is referred to as the "awakened one." *Buddhi* is where we find those much sought after faculties of wisdom, knowledge, reflection, witnessing, and discernment. *Buddhi*, unlike *manas*, is able to see outside the confines of time and space, i.e., *buddhi* has access to information the senses don't have. *Buddhi* is the call we each feel to grow, to transcend, and to be more than we are.

The ability to engage the witness opens up new possibilities. The mind is able to observe the outer world, i.e., it can watch the sensory exchange (and any knee-jerk reactions that might accompany the exchange) as it is occurring. The mind can also observe the inner world, i.e., it can watch any sensations of tightening or relaxing occurring in the body as the exchange happens. And the mind can observe itself, i.e., it can watch how it manages the whole process.

The ability to observe (witness) the mind creates distance from the mind and leaves us with the experience that we are not the mind itself, but something else. Rather than identifying with our minds, we begin to see that our minds, like the bodies we inhabit, can be nourished, trained, and cared for in a manner that will allow for a life of potency and joy.

Even while *manas* (importer and exporter of data) and the enticement of the senses can call us to get lost in the outer world; even while *ahamkara* (I-maker) can make us feel small, separate, and protective of our identity; *buddhi* (the witness / higher mind) is quietly calling us to wholeness by providing us the means to explore the more subtle aspects of our being and to know that there is more than what the senses and ego show us.

When I broke my arm, there was enough displacement of the bone ends to require surgery and the support of a plate and screws to put the two broken pieces of bone back in place. A few weeks after surgery, I observed the first x-rays taken to see how the bone was healing. The x-rays showed a new growth of tiny filaments on the end of each break. I was seeing the initial process of my bone healing as the two broken ends began to reach out for each other seeking unity and wholeness again. In a similar fashion, the mind is always seeking to be healed and whole, and it is *buddhi* whispering that desire to us.

Reflection: Explore the function known as *buddhi*, the higher mind. Do you experience any soft whisperings within you? Is there something inside gently urging you to grow, expand, and to reach for a greater sense of wholeness?

Reflection: Notice the ability the mind has to watch itself. Choose something to engage in (dishes, eating, walking). Do the activity without watching your mind and then do it watching your mind. What changes in your experience when you watch your mind?

The Thinking Process

It is important to remember that the functions of the mind are not separate parts but co-arise as a unified mind, and the whole process of thinking is influenced by the individual storehouse of personal conditioning, whether conscious or unconscious, with awareness or without awareness.

The mind draws a boundary of separation, creating an inner world (me) and an outer world (them, it). It processes information from the outer world, decides what to do with it, and then acts on the outer world. This exchange happens through the sense organs and the electrical/chemical processes of the brain. But how does this information get interpreted? Through the subjective conditioning stored in the mind. In other words, information goes in (*manas*), it feels personal (*ahamkara* / ego), it gets routed through the storehouse of our stories, conditioning, and beliefs (*chitta*), and then we react or respond accordingly.

We can look at life from the unexamined, conditioned mind alone, or we can ask what shapes our thinking and actions.

We don't just take in information. We think about it, add feelings from memory, and report the information to *buddhi*. If the functions of the mind are not acting in a coordinated manner and ego is not kept in check, *manas* receives skewed directions or acts on its own. Simply put, unless we have begun a path of self-awareness, in which we use *buddhi* (the higher mind) to see and operate independently of our conditioning, we continue to interpret and react according to our conditioning.

The limits of our conditioning are not bad in themselves; as long as we know they are limited, they can be a solid base for experience, humility, and growth. Knowing that our ignorance causes suffering for ourselves and others can be a powerful impetus for spiritual reflection and discipline. Being hungry to know what we don't know can pull us towards greater truths.

But when we don't understand that what seems real to us is vastly incomplete, we feel the need to protect it by whatever means necessary. When we are busy protecting and attaining, we don't have time to question the long-term results of our actions. We may cling to achievements so tightly that in the process of achieving we lose our health. We may value being right so highly that in the insistence to be right, we lose important relationships. We may value having things so greatly that in the process we accumulate far more than we need causing hardship and deprivation for others.

The point is, we can look at life from the unexamined, conditioned mind alone, which often leads to the suffering produced by narcissism, self-interest, anxiety, and going to extreme lengths to protect what we own. Or we can ask what it is that shapes our thinking and actions. Asking this question leads to curiosity about our own conditioning and the quest to know who we really are.

Some of the conditioning, trauma, and other undigested

experiences sit in our conscious awareness. But much of the narrative and experience that hold power over our lives was set in motion before we had conceptual understanding; they sit in the very tissues of our bodies as visceral experience without language. They direct our lives, and we don't know it or know why because they are unconscious.

Have you ever left a yoga class feeling so peaceful you knew nothing could ever upset you? And yet, two minutes later a car pulls out in front of you and you find yourself blurting out expletives? It happened so quickly that you never had time to think about it. After you've calmed down you wonder what just happened. This is the power our conditioning and unresolved experiences hold over us.

The mind seeks to heal these undigested experiences that burden it. It seeks to expand the narrative, to let go of what it is clinging to, and to stop resisting what it is avoiding. It seeks to rest in its innate tranquil state, free of roaming tendencies and the conditioning that entangles it. How this happens is the subject of the next section.

Reflection: What is your experience of thinking? Of all the different possibilities for thought to take, why are you thinking the thoughts you're thinking right now? Do you believe your thoughts? Why or why not?

Reflection: Write a letter to your mind. Write knowing your mind is your best friend, and your worst enemy. It is your most powerful advocate, and your trickiest adversary. After you have written the letter, reflect on what you have written.

Mind Practices ~ VEDANTA MODEL

Manas ~ SENSORY INPUT & EXPORT
☒ Cut down sensory input by 1/3
    (technology, noise, sugar, caffeine)
☒ Guard the first and last hour of your day
    (guard it with quiet and ease)
☒ Slow down and do one thing at a time

Ahamkara ~ THE "I" MAKER (EGO)
✾ Read sacred scripture
✾ Be part of something that is in service to others
✾ Use as few "I, me and mine" as possible

Chitta ~ STOREHOUSE OF ALL SENSORY DATA, MEMORY,
    CONDITIONING, AND BELIEFS
✾ Meditate, journal, reflect daily
✾ Trace all disturbances back to your conditioning
✾ Cultivate a virtue (generosity, gratitude, compassion...)

Buddhi ~ WITNESS/DISCERNER
❀ Practice listening to your intuition
❀ Practice witnessing and observing
❀ Practice the ability to see cause & effect

Practice & Nonattachment

THE POWER

Whether we are brushing our teeth,
interacting with family members,
or sitting on our cushion,
mastering the mind requires diligence
to both practice and nonattachment.

I like to imagine what it was like to be those first yogis. Of course, I have no idea, but the act of imagination is an interesting one. Without the abundance of books and accomplished teachers to guide them, I wonder what people did before access to so much wisdom was available. Were they guided by their strong desire to know more, their immense curiosity, their willingness to observe and experiment? Or perhaps all of these led to their accomplished learning.

In my imagination, their desire to understand the "how" of things caused them to become keen observers of life. They used their own lives and bodies as a laboratory for exploration. And once they had assessed the situation, naming what they found with their understanding of the *kleshas* and their study of the mind, they had a lot of information.

But they didn't stop there. Once the yogis understood the workings of their minds, their conditioning, their preferences, and what a mess people could make of life, they were led to ask more questions. Questions like: If this is how things are, is it possible to get on the "good" side of things? Is it possible to teach my mind to do something else? Can future suffering be avoided? How would I do that?

Yogis asked themselves questions like: If this is how things are, is it possible to get on the "good" side of things? Is it possible to teach my mind to do something else? Can future suffering be avoided? How would I do that?

Aware of the many uncontrollable factors in the outer world, they turned inward, to the place where they had absolute autonomy, to see if a kind of paradise could be created and sustained in their inner world, and to see what impact their inner world might have on the outer world. And they worked with their minds. Because they had realized they had the power to witness their own thoughts and actions, they could notice and reflect on what bound them to affliction. They could watch and they could choose. This, they realized, was where change could happen.

Whatever their process, one thing they must have known for sure: if they didn't do anything different, nothing would change. So they experimented; they discovered what worked for them, and then they shared their knowledge.

Whatever their process, one thing they must have known for sure: if they didn't do anything different, nothing would change. They needed to find a new way to be with their conditioning so it was not in charge of their minds, hijacking their nervous systems, and controlling their happiness. So they experimented; they discovered what worked for them and what didn't. And then they shared their knowledge and their new plan for the mind.

Nirodha ~ *A NEW PLAN FOR THE MIND*

Nirodha changes everything: how we use our minds, the choices we make, the actions we take, and the quality of our lives.

To grasp the power of this word, we return to Yoga Sutra 1:2 where Patanjali uses only three words to define yoga: *chitta* (for the mind), *vrittis* (for the mind's tendency to roam), and *nirodha* (the key word that frees the mind). In English, *nirodha* gets translated as restraint, control, cessation, arresting, and mastery by Sanskrit scholars.

When Patanjali defines yoga, he is unequivocally stating that yoga is the practice and ultimate attainment of a mind that is not at the mercy of roaming, nor limited by the dictates of its conditioning. When I reflect on the immense power of my mind to think and do what it wants, this definition seems almost miraculous. Yet, this is not just one man's personal definition. Rather, it is the common experiential understanding of yoga as it has been practiced for thousands of years by thousands of practitioners. This is a definition tested by time, numbers, and success.

> Yoga is the practice and ultimate attainment of a mind that is not at the mercy of roaming nor limited by the dictates of its conditioning.

Nirodha's effectiveness is based on two equally important components: *abhyasa,* or practice, and *vairagya,* or nonattachment (Yoga Sutra 1:12). One without the other is a guarantee that we will fail at this arduous task of training the mind. Whether we are brushing our teeth, interacting with family members, or sitting on our cushion, mastering the mind requires diligence to both practice and nonattachment.

Mastering the mind is accomplished through practice (*abhyasa*) + nonattachment (*vairagya*). These two components, working together, are a declaration that we have the power to choose where we put our attention, and we have the power to let go of the things that hold us captive.

We will explore both of these aspects of *nirodha* (mastery) in following sections, but briefly put, practice (*abhyasa*) addresses the mind's wandering by training the mind to peacefully stay in one place. Nonattachment (*vairagya*) addresses the mind's oscillating pattern by loosening our tendency to cling and resist. Together, practice and nonattachment are a declaration that we have the power to choose where we put our attention, and we have the power to let go of the things that hold us captive. Together, these two components go right to the heart of our mind's bondage to the *kleshas* and return it to its inherent clear and tranquil nature.

Some 600 years prior to the compilation of the Yoga Sutra, similar words were spoken in the Bhagavad Gita. The teacher Krishna tells his student Arjuna that the mind can be brought to a place where it is as still as the flame of a candle when there is no wind. Arjuna, perhaps astonished by such a statement, declares that trying to control the mind is like trying to control the wind. To which Krishna responds that Arjuna is correct, but nevertheless, the mind can be conquered through practice and nonattachment (Bhagavad Gita 6:19, 34, 35).

Let's look in turn at these two powerful actions that, when paired, can tame the mind and bring it to a place where it is as still as the flame of a candle when there is no wind.

Abhyasa ~ PRACTICE

What do you cherish most? Is it your family? Your health? Your success? Your image? There is no "right" answer; this is a personal question to be answered by each of us individually. How we answer reveals what is uppermost in importance to us, in other words, where we put our attention…or at least attempt to.

Attention is getting more press these days. We hear phrases like "attention economy" and "attention merchants," a reminder that advertisers get paid big bucks to take advantage of our weak minds. As we get sucked into social media, internet surfing, and unintentional online shopping, we may be tempted to ask, "Whose mind is this?"

With the ease and newness of so much information at our fingertips, this may seem like a new problem for humans. Yet if we look at the ancient yoga texts, we find that the power to put the mind where we want to and keep it there was a problem for ancient spiritual seekers, as well as it is for us today.

The problem has been, and is, the mind's proclivity to roam, to be captured by conditioning, by preferences, by outside sensory stimulation, and yes, by attention merchants. Practice then, is about who owns our attention. Practice is a vigilance over the mind's attention and the effort to stay focused. Practice is a declaration: My mind is one of the most precious things I have, and I want to harness its potential.

Practice is not about what we don't want or about trying to make things better. Practice has nothing to do with self-improvement, feeling worthy and deserving, being enough, fixing ourselves, or anything that has to do with attempts to improve our *klesha* experience.

Our minds are caught in a cluttered, roaming pattern. We have to do something or we will remain prisoners of this pattern and its consequences. That "something" is to master these roaming tendencies by training the mind to stay steady. Practice, then, is everything we do to stabilize the mind. It is the effort to master the roaming tendencies by bringing the mind to a steady peaceful flow.

Have you ever witnessed a calm lake, so still it takes your breath away with its peacefulness? Have you noticed how the calmness creates clarity? You can see all the way to the bottom of the lake. You can distinctly see the algae and fish alive in the water. But if the wind comes up or you begin skipping stones across the water, things change. The turbulence from the disturbance creates murkiness and distortion. You can no longer see clearly, and the bottom of the lake is hidden from view.

> Practice = the effort to bring the mind to a steady peaceful flow; the effort to stabilize the mind.

Such is the state of our minds. Our "clinging to" and "pushing away" is like a constant wind causing waves of disturbance in the mind. It is like skipping rocks in our mind without letting up. We can't see reality clearly; we can't see others clearly; we can't see ourselves clearly.

Practice is the effort to quiet the mind. Stop the winds of clinging and resisting. Stop throwing the rocks of reactions. Counter the habit of oscillating with the practice of one-pointedness. Create a stable mind, and clarity will follow.

Stability of mind means we choose what our mind entertains. We focus where we want to focus and keep our attention where we want to keep it, without being sidetracked. We do this with intention and attention, two innate gifts that get hijacked by the roaming tendencies.

The practice of bringing a scattered mind to one place and keeping it there can be discouraging; it is easy on some days to feel that the practice isn't working, or perhaps even making things worse. But that is why it is called practice. Practice is both the mirror that allows us to see the current state of our minds and it is the vehicle that leads us to a different mind.

I began my yoga practice mostly as a course of self-improvement. I was looking for something I knew was missing in my life. Even though I felt wonderful at the end of class, there was always that pressure, always something more I needed, whether it was props, outfits, additional classes or books or just to be more skilled and knowledgeable, there was always the next thing. I could only understand yoga and its practice through my narrative, one of never-ending attainment and self-improvement. This was not a failure of yoga or of my teachers, it was a failure of my narrative to grasp the profoundness of practice itself.

I also thought my yoga practice sat outside the rest of my life. It had its own separate category and place in my daily schedule. I knew I was not alone in this view of practice when I began to receive emails from people who had read the *Yamas & Niyamas* book and wondered how they were supposed to add this ethical practice to their already over-scheduled lives.

But that's the thing, practice requires not only its own concentrated time on the mat and on the cushion, but it can be done all the time. We can bring all of our awareness to the task at hand, keep watch over our thoughts and, when needed, coax them towards kindness, and observe the ways our conditioning limits us. This is available to us all the time because our mind goes everywhere we go.

If the lived experience of the *kleshas* (afflictions) is:	Then *abhyasa* (practice) is designed to bring a new experience:
Oscillating in the ups and downs.	Stability of mind.
Controlled by the pull of the senses and reactions to the outer world.	An inner source of lasting pleasure.
Emotionally entangled in fear, greed, and self-centeredness.	Unwavering trust, courage, and joy.

Besides bringing stability to the mind, practice helps us find a right relationship with the senses so that we can enjoy them without being controlled by them. To return to the Katha Upanishad and the image of a chariot driven by ten horses where the chariot represents the physical body and the horses represent the ten senses, when the reins are held loosely, the horses (ten senses) can go wherever they want.

Practice is both the mirror that allows us to see the current state of our minds and it is the vehicle that leads us to a different mind.

Anything that looks inviting can take them off the path and onto rough terrain. In the process, the chariot (our body) gets bumped and scratched and in need of repairs. But when the reins are controlled by the clarity and discernment of a stable mind, the horses are kept on the path, and the ride is smooth.

For those of us caught in the unquenchable pull of the senses, this image is not hard to grasp. How many of us can feel the wornness of our bodies from the excess of food, drink, work, or technology? How many of us sit in the clutter of our excess, even as we grasp to buy the next thing? It is so easy to let down our guard just a little, just this once…and the horses are off and running.

Practice is having a steady grasp on the reins of sensory pleasures so that we stay on the path. But how do we do this when the outside world tantalizes and taunts us with its fleeting pleasures? How do we do this in a world of overwhelming sensory stimulation? How do we control the reins of our desires when our habitual response is to satisfy them?

To this, Patanjali suggests that we begin to explore and become familiar with the inner world, the subjective world particular to each self. The inner world is inhabited with our unique conditioning, beliefs, experiences, memory, and imagination. We explore and become familiar with the inner world through silence, through reflection, through listening, and through meditation. To explore and become familiar with the inner world we quiet the senses and gain skill in different ways of knowing such as witnessing, awareness, presence, and mindfulness.

It is in the time we spend in the inner world that we learn discernment and clarity. We begin to see through the momentary promises of sensory objects. This gives us the skill to see our daily choices played out before us. The invitation for pizza and a movie at 10pm carries with it not just the pleasure of an evening, but

> We become familiar with the inner world through silence, reflection, listening, and meditation. We gain skill in different ways of knowing such as witnessing, awareness, presence, and mindfulness.

the aftermath of bloating and lethargy the next morning. We may choose the pizza, we may not, but we do it from a place of knowing the cost. That in itself is significant.

As we spend periods of time in silence, reflection, prayer, and meditation, we may begin to hear a different message than the one we have become familiar with. It is a message that begins to source us in an inner strength. It might sound something like this:

> The outer world says: you are your gender, your class, your personality, your talents;
> The inner world says: this is just packaging, keep looking deeper.
>
> The outer world says: hurry, faster;
> The inner world says: slowly, slowly.
>
> The outer world says: get more, more;
> The inner world says: let go, need less.
>
> The outer world says: you aren't perfect; you need this and a little of this, and a lot of that;
> The inner world says: you already have everything you need inside.
>
> The outer world says: people should notice you;
> The inner world says: notice others.
>
> The outer world says: your life should be perfect;
> The inner world says: be perfect in your life.

Besides stabilizing the mind and finding a right relationship with the senses, practice (*abhyasa*) directly addresses our negative emotions and replaces them with more noble virtues.

The importance of this cannot be overemphasized. As our minds become more one-pointed, they become more potent. We have only to reflect on the amazing inventions and creative endeavors throughout history and into the present day to grasp what these minds are capable of. We can also be aware of both the life-giving and destructive outcomes of these great feats of mind.

Feelings of selfishness, fear, loneliness, hatred, and anger, to name a few, are all indicators that our thoughts are bound to the misunderstandings of the *kleshas*. When these negative thoughts harass us, Patanjali tells us in Yoga Sutra 2:33, we should encourage counteracting thoughts.

When our mind is filled with any negative thought, this is the time for practice. It's as if a water pipe in our home has broken and water is spewing all over ruining the carpets and furniture. The only way to stop the damage is to stop the flow of water. Likewise, when our mind is engaged in negative tendencies the only way to stop the damage to our body/mind is to replace the negative flow of thought with a nourishing thought.

> When our mind is filled with any negative thought, this is the time for practice. The only way to stop the damage is to stop the flow of negative thoughts by replacing them with a flow of nourishing thoughts.

In case we are short on ideas of what these nourishing, counteracting thoughts might be, Patanjali is ready with suggestions. In Yoga Sutra 1:33, he tells us that "Transparency of mind comes by embracing an attitude of friendliness, compassion, happiness, and non-judgment toward those who are happy, miserable, virtuous, and non-virtuous" (Tigunait, p. 161). Friendliness, compassion, happiness, and non-judgment are the highest qualities available to human nature and the resting place for peaceful minds.

Embrace an Attitude of:
Friendliness toward those who are happy; Compassion toward those who are miserable; Happiness toward those who are virtuous; Nonjudgment toward those who are nonvirtuous.

Similar words were spoken by the Apostle Paul in the New Testament when he wrote these words to the congregation at Philippi, "Finally, beloved, whatever is true, whatever is honorable, whatever is just, whatever is pure, whatever is pleasing, whatever is commendable, if there is any excellence and if there is anything worthy of praise, think about these things" (Philippians 4:8, New Revised Standard Version).

Schadenfreude is a word I have recently become familiar with. Coming from two words that respectively mean harm and joy, it describes the joy a person can feel when they witness the misery or misfortune of another. Lest we think we are immune from this kind of cynical joy, studies have shown this tendency exists in children as young as 24 months.

Whether we find ourselves fighting or denying the monsters of hatred and cruelty inside of us or outside of us, it is important to remember to foster what we want, not fight against what we don't want. We are filling the mind with noble attitudes until all the negative tendencies spill out because they no longer have room in our mind.

Reflection: In what way(s) would your practice change if you thought of practice as stabilizing your mind?

Reflection: Are there places in your life where the senses are in control of you? Describe the experience. Can you relate to the image of the chariot and horses in the Katha Upanishad? In what way?

Reflection: This week, when you are harassed by negative thoughts, encourage counteracting thoughts. What do you notice?

How to Practice

In my neighborhood, the homes are built close together, and almost every home has at least one dog. Living in such close proximity to the daily activities of the neighborhood, I have, over time, come to find the relationship between owner and dog to be not only entertaining, but instructive.

Some dogs seem totally untrained and not about to respond to their owner's repeated commands; their will is their own. Others seem submissive with a lowered head and absent spirit, the unwilling victims of cruelty. They are well behaved, but it comes from fear of their owners.

Then there are those rare dogs that go unleashed; they are free, yet training and love have captured their allegiance. They are paradoxically fully obedient, yet full of spark and life. The relationship between dog and owner is one of harmony and synchronicity. As I watch this litany of training and its results, the importance of how we train our minds becomes apparent.

The undisciplined mind is like a new puppy, full of energy and lack of direction. We can let the mind stay undisciplined, hoping someday it will "grow out of it." We can treat the mind harshly, shaming it and filling it with images of what we don't want it to do. Or we can treat our mind tenderly, yet firmly, to be a faithful and loving mind. Patanjali suggests the latter.

Following his explanation of practice, Patanjali gives three guidelines for how we are to practice. He tells us that practice should be uninterrupted, done for a long period of time, and infused with devotion (Yoga Sutra 1:14). These three things create a momentum that turns practice into a transformative force.

Practice Should Be:
Uninterrupted; Done for a long period of time; Infused with devotion.

Practice should be uninterrupted. This seems obvious. After all, we can't just potty train a new puppy once a week and expect it to be trained. Teaching a puppy to relieve itself outside takes constant vigilance, especially until the puppy begins to catch on and asks to be let out. Beautiful gardens do not create and maintain themselves. They need to be watered, weeded, and lovingly cared for on a consistent basis. I couldn't do my arm exercises only when I felt like it and expect to have a fully functioning arm after the cast was removed. If we want our minds to do one thing and they are used to doing another, there is some uninterrupted attention required on our parts.

Uninterrupted practice does not mean that we need to meditate or do postures or breath practices twenty-four hours a day every day. It means that whether we are engaged in these specific practices or doing the laundry, we are paying attention to our minds. When they start to wander towards worry or negative thoughts or harsh judgments, we gently and firmly bring them back to thoughts of a higher quality. When our minds are jumping all over, distracted and unfocused, we firmly and gently bring them back to the breath or to the task at hand. When our minds are dull and cloudy, we check the quality of our food, sleep, and activities.

> The importance of practice is that we keep bringing the mind back to where we want it to be.

The importance of practice is that we keep bringing the mind back to where we want it to be. We notice it has been hijacked yet again, and we patiently bring it back. We don't practice because we are good at something; we practice because we want to be good at something.

Practice should be done for a long period of time. We can click a button on Amazon and have whatever we want delivered the next day. We can have mail overnighted. We can watch almost any movie we want immediately on our device. We can contact someone around the world and hear back from them within seconds. A culture of instantaneous gratification means we don't have to wait.

Technology has made many things possible, including access to learning about yoga, about the brain, about self-love, and about changing our habits. But our instant access to so much has not changed the "long period of time" part of practice. We may have instant access to knowledge, but not to experiential knowing. There is a persistency to practice, a need to be patient without being sluggish. It was true for Patanjali, and it is true for us.

At the age of 45, my dad had a massive heart attack. It should have killed him; instead he was home after a month in the hospital, weak and bed-ridden. Recovery was a long process. For many weeks all he could manage was a slow and tedious walk to the bedroom door and back to bed. Then he managed a daily walk down the hallway. Eventually he was in the living area and then outdoors walking on the sidewalk. In what seemed like a miracle, I watched my dad over a long period of time reach his goal of a brisk two and a half mile daily walk. It was a walk he continued into his eighties. His patient, daily practice led to decades of vibrant living.

Practice should be infused with devotion. I often hear people described as being devoted to their children, devoted to their work, or devoted to a particular cause. People get talked about in this way because there is no question about where their quality time goes, where their priority lies, or what brings a sparkle to their eyes. There is an obvious quality to the satisfying dedication that a person gives to the object of their devotion. Devotion connotes a sense of awe, reverence, great love, loyalty, and profound dedication. It is there because we feel that thing is worthy of our time and energy.

How we practice determines the quality of our practice, and the quality of our practice influences its transformative power.

How we practice determines the quality of our practice, and the quality of our practice influences its transformative power. We are engaged in a practice that takes us from suffering to

121

innate joy. We are engaged in a practice that takes us from ignorance to wisdom. We are engaged in a practice to know fully who we are, the truth of reality, and the source behind it all. What could be more awe-inspiring, more intriguing, and more important than the opportunity to practice? What could elicit more devotion than practice? Remember, we are not trying to "fix" ourselves, rather practice is done from the hunger to heal and be whole.

> Practice is done from the hunger to heal and be whole.

The Sufi mystics believe that we are born with ten thousand veils separating us from the truth. Practice that is uninterrupted, done for a long period of time, and infused with devotion is what brings the clarity and discernment needed to penetrate these veils.

Reflection: What attitude do you bring to your practice? Is it one of obligation? Is it the goal to check it off your "to do" list? Is it from a deep longing or hunger? What is it that brings you to your practice?

Reflection: Patanjali states that practice should be "infused with devotion." What does that mean to you? In what way(s) is your practice "infused with devotion"?

Reflection: Using the analogy of someone training their puppy, how do you personally train your mind? Do you yell at it? Do you beat yourself up verbally? Do you let your mind roam where it wants to? Are you firm but loving? What kind of mind owner are you?

What to Practice

Watching sports movies, especially of high school teams with a discouraging losing streak, is something I enjoy. The plot is always similar: a new coach comes in and immediately takes the team back to the basics. Mumbling and groaning, the team runs continuous laps and endless practice drills, all the while wondering what this has to do with winning a game.

It's inspiring to watch as, over time, the team grows in confidence, and they begin to understand why the laps and drills are so important. They solidify as a team, along with growing personally, and their effort soon finds them on a winning streak. A good coach knows you can't take a team who is used to losing and turn them into winners without the endurance built by running and the ability built by drills.

In similar fashion, Patanjali knows he is coaching a losing team. The roaming tendencies have created dis-ease in our bodies, mental agitation in our minds, poor choices in our lives, and obstacles to our transformation. All these aspects need to be addressed. And, with the 8-limbed path, Patanjali has the winning plan to foster a body in ease, a mind flowing peacefully, and a life lived in harmony. This is the environment that opens the door to victory.

Returning to Patanjali's definition of yoga as mastery over the roaming tendencies of the mind, it is meditation that sits at the heart of such mastery. It is in meditation that the mind is turned inward to look at itself and its conditioned habits and

123

beliefs. It is in meditation that the senses are pulled inward to rest, allowing for a different way to receive information. And it is in meditation that the mind becomes stabilized, producing a clarity that allows us to see what we can't see when the mind is busy.

But meditation isn't something we can just do on demand; it takes preparation and getting all of ourselves lined up, content, and on board with this unique process of being still. And so we are given the 8-limbed path, eight steps to prepare and practice keeping the mind peaceful and steady while lessening the grip of our habitual clinging and resisting tendency. Note that although these eight limbs go from the grosser (more tangible) to the subtler parts of our life, they are circular, not linear, and they are worthy of our attention at all times.

The 8-Limbed Path

Yamas ~ the restraints: nonviolence, truthfulness, nonstealing, nonexcess, nonpossessiveness
Niyamas ~ the observances: purity, contentment, self-discipline, self-study, surrender
Asana ~ the body's posturing
Pranayama ~ our relationship with cosmic life force
Pratyahara ~ pulling in of the senses
Dharana ~ concentration
Dhyana ~ meditation
Samadhi ~ absorption

These eight limbs address all levels and activities of our being, and, when done well, each limb leads to the success of the other limbs. They bring about harmony in the whole system, bringing integrity to relationships, comfort to the body, ease to the breath, and an awareness turned inward that allows us to quietly watch the mind in action.

The question is: how do we take the essence of each limb, hold it in the light of our particular imbalance, and shape a personal practice that creates mastery over the roaming tendencies? How do we create a lifestyle conducive to knowing ourselves? How do we get all the parts of the psyche online?

Limb 1: Yamas ~ THE RESTRAINTS

I remember an incident from a weeklong retreat I attended many years ago. It was towards the end of the week, the lectures had been dense, we were all weary and brain dead, when one of the students excitedly exclaimed, "Oh, I get it; yoga is about three things:
 1. Don't disturb yourself.
 2. Don't disturb others.
 3. See #1!"

Her outburst was a much-needed relief to the detailed learning of the week. Together we broke out in collective laughter, recognizing a deep truth to the simplicity of her exclamation. Perhaps at its core, yoga is about becoming "undisturbed, undisturbing, and undisturbable."

The plan for training a mind that flows peacefully begins with an ethical system, because, well let's face it, what could provide more cause for disturbance than our relationships? And isn't everything a relationship? We have a relationship with the past and the future, with the living and the dead, with those like us and those unlike us, with those we know and those we don't. We have a relationship with climate, with politics, with religion, with the Divine. And we have a relationship with ourselves.

All of these relationships carry a fluctuating degree of clinging and resisting, of emotional highs and emotional lows. Depending on the particulars of the moment, they evoke in us anything from compassion to downright rage. They are the stuff the roaming tendencies love to feed on. To combat disturbances in our relationships, five practices are given to us in this first limb: nonviolence, truthfulness, nonstealing, nonexcess, and nonpossessiveness.

The impact of practicing these guidelines cannot be overemphasized. Have you ever had a fight with someone who is dear to you? I have. And for many hours afterwards, my mind is in turbulence. I am replaying the fight over and over and wondering how that person could have done such a thing...or I am wondering how I could have said such a thing to them.

Or have you ever told someone you would do something with them, but you really didn't want to? Those instances for me are again times I play the scenario over and over wondering how I can get out of it or miserably looking forward to having to do it. In both of these instances, disturbance rules.

The word *yamas* translates as restraints. It's as if in this first limb of the path, Patanjali is saying to us: *Look, you don't have to be like Gandhi or Mother Theresa right off the bat. But could you please just try to stop making things worse than they are! Restrain yourself from the disturbance caused (to others and yourself) when you do harm, or withhold the truth, or steal, or when you over-indulge, or when you try to possess.*

Restraint is an interesting word. We had a neighbor who was abusive to his wife. In one particularly violent episode, the police were summoned. They handcuffed the husband and hauled him away. He was then given a restraining order that forbade him from being on the property near his wife for six months. In much the same manner, perhaps Patanjali is issuing us a restraining order in this first limb of the path to keep us from causing any more disturbance.

We have most likely witnessed an ambulance arrive at a critical situation, the EMT's carefully placing the person at risk on a cot, and steadily carrying them to the ambulance, where they are whisked away for further help. Often, restraints are used to keep the person in place, especially when an IV is applied. In this case, the restraint is used to keep the person aligned with the life-saving measures in place. In much the same manner, perhaps Patanjali is putting restraints on us as a life-saving measure.

Both of these images support me when I'm feeling angry or acting in excess or out of greed. I can almost visualize

Patanjali restraining my hands to keep me from creating waves of disturbance. At other times, I imagine Patanjali is carefully restraining me on a cot, intravenously infusing me with the life-giving elixir of right relationship and helping me to see that nothing is worth sacrificing my equanimity.

Reflection: What does harmony feel like in your body? Where do you feel it? What does being out of harmony feel like in your body? Where do you feel it?

Limb 2: Niyamas ~ THE OBSERVANCES

With the *yamas*, Patanjali has clarified for us what a diet of junk food for the mind is. Violence, failing to tell the truth, stealing, indulgence, possessiveness, these things clog the arteries of our mind. They cause a toxic environment in which the roaming tendencies can flourish.

With the *niyamas*, Patanjali lays out a healthy diet plan for the mind that unclogs the pathways, purifies the environment, and gives the mind a resting place to peacefully flow. But much like replacing the empty calories of a candy bar with the nourishing qualities of broccoli, the observances may not seem all that appealing at first. After all, disturbance stirs up the emotions and often leads to a sense of righteous indignation, a feeling we can take false pride in. Our minds have grown accustomed to turbulent thoughts and emotions, and the observances appear bland and boring to a mind used to more exciting activity. It may take a while for the mind to fully appreciate the seemingly less attractive qualities of a simpler, nourishing, thought-diet.

There are five practices that comprise the second limb. Purity, which asks us to simplify our lives; contentment, which asks us to allow life to be as it is; self-discipline, which asks us to take responsible action; self-study, which asks us to look at our involvement in disturbance; and surrender, which reminds us that everything is not about us. As we begin to focus on these observances, the mind becomes interested in the process and less enamored with the false appeal of chaos. The mind is beginning to enjoy its new diet of thoughts and to relish the calm it is bringing.

Our minds have grown accustomed to turbulent thoughts and emotions. It may take a while for the mind to fully appreciate the qualities of a simpler, nourishing, thought-diet.

I. K. Taimni, in his commentary on the Yoga Sutras calls the *yamas & niyamas* a "very drastic ethical code" stating that, "The main object of this relentless ethical code [the *yamas & niyamas*] is to eliminate completely all mental and emotional disturbances which characterize the life of an ordinary human being." He goes on to say, "And, as long as these disturbances continue to affect the mind it is useless to undertake the more systematic and advanced practice of *Yoga*" (Taimni, p. 209).

When I have shared the above quote in various teaching situations, it is met with mixed reactions. Some participants agree entirely, others react with adamant disagreement. Regardless of whether we agree with Taimni or not, the question of why Patanjali begins with an ethical system or why he dedicates one fourth of the path of mastery to ethical behavior is worthy of our contemplation.

Reflection: The word ethics comes from the Greek word *ethos* and carries a meaning of the "as usuals" of life. This meaning encourages us to look at what is the "as usual" in our relational stance (self and other). Is it one that brings discord or tranquility?

Limb 3: Asana ~ THE BODY'S POSTURING

It's hard not to admire a body that has mastered *asana*. The fluidity, strength, balance, and ease in which each position is assumed and effortlessly held is mesmerizing. Personally, my body has never come close to attaining that kind of mastery; I am more of an *asana* want-to-be.

People come to this third limb of the practice with bodies of different capabilities. Some suffer from arthritis, some from injury, others from chronic illness, slipped discs, others from paralysis, and still others with the fitness of a marathon runner. Some come having sat at a desk all day; others come dead on their feet from a physically demanding job. Some of us try to force our bodies into places they are not ready to go; others of us give up all together.

Mastery of the mind does not come from force or from giving up, but from an understanding of how this limb moves the mind from disturbance to tranquility. At its essence, *asana* means "seat" and that, Patanjali says, means being both comfortable and steady, the goal being to attain a comfortable, steady position that we can hold easily and effortlessly for longer and longer periods of time. This is true mastery of the body.

One of my favorite cartoons is of the "Boneless Chicken Ranch" in *The Far Side* series by Gary Larson. This particular cartoon depicts a scene with many chickens scattered about the ranch, each flopped in a stagnant position because they have nothing to support them. It is comical, but also instructive. In *asana* we are looking for the right amount of effort, just enough to do what is required for the task at hand, but not more than is necessary.

Asana postures are designed to align our bodies in a fashion that brings ease and functionality to both movement and stillness. They offer an opening to knotted places, a strengthening of internal stability, the grace of integration, and the surety of balance. All of these enable the body to sit with greater comfort and stability for longer periods of time.

> *Asana* is a "posturing" stance, an invitation to create a body that can move through life with greater ease and steadiness, no matter what our circumstances.

It is easy to think of *asana* as the yoga postures themselves, but more than postures, this limb is a "posturing," a stance, an invitation to create a body that can move through life with greater ease and steadiness, no matter what our circumstances.

131

That means the how's, what's, and when's we eat and sleep matter. Our ability to nourish, replenish, eliminate toxins, and maintain our body's health, balance, and endurance matters.

All of this matters because a body that doesn't get enough movement equals a mind that is foggy and stupefied. A body that eats excessively equals a mind that is bloated. A body that doesn't get enough rest equals a mind that is exhausted. A body that is not comfortable and steady equals a mind that is free to roam. Everything we do to strengthen, nourish, and bring ease to the body directly affects the mind.

What can we do (or stop doing) that will bring more ease and steadiness to our body? How much comfort and steadiness is possible for this body today, in this moment, within the context of our circumstances? "Steady and comfortable," Patanjali tells us, leads to "effortless effort." What would it be like to move through life with this kind of posturing? And how would our minds be different if we did?

Try this simple practice: Sit upright in a chair without slouching your shoulders, sinking into the chair, or propping yourself up. Can you find that "just right place" where you are steady and comfortable? Could you sit like this for an hour or more? Can you find the feeling of effortless effort? Why or why not?

Begin to take this practice of simultaneous steadiness and comfort to various activities such as brushing your teeth, getting dressed, walking, etc.

Reflection: Notice the amount of effort you put into things this week. What is happening in your mind when you are exerting yourself? Can you build resilience by softening your approach? What do you notice?

Limb 4: Pranayama ~ OUR RELATIONSHIP WITH LIFE FORCE

Breath is the great connector and equalizer. Breath connects us to the green beings that live in our homes, outside our homes, and in the far corners of the world. It connects us to each other. It connects the inner world and the outer world, our discerning power with sensory knowledge. Our emotions dance with it; our nervous systems reflect it.

Breath has always been there for us. In our suffering, our anger, our joy, our aging, breath breathes us. We may receive the breath by assisting, controlling, holding, aborting, or forcing it. But it doesn't change, we do. Breath does not fail us; we fail the breath.

> Breath is the great connector and equalizer. Breath connects us to the earth and to each other. It connects the inner world and the outer world. It connects our discerning power with sensory knowledge.

We cut down prime forests as if our lungs were a separate entity; we release toxins into the air in the name of continued luxury; we spew words of anger and judgment as if the impact was inconsequential. And then we breathe this air. We breathe our own personal and collective human failings.

We plant trees, protect forests, choose simplicity over extravagance, speak words of kindness and nourishment. And then we breathe this air. We breathe our own personal and collective human capabilities.

We come into this world and become breathing beings. We leave this world when breathing stops. Every day, every hour, every minute, from birth to death, breath continually enters and leaves our bodies. How we receive it; how we release it matters. We contribute to the harmony and disharmony in ourselves and outside ourselves with every breath.

A disturbed breath reflects a nervous system that is stressed, a mind that is caught in the roaming tendencies, and a contribution to self and others that is dissonant. A slow, smooth, easy flowing breath reflects the opposite. Through breath practices, awareness of this process is heightened, resistance is softened, and ease and steadiness of breath are increased.

As our relationship with breath deepens, we become aware of a more subtle presence within the breath called *prana*, the life force itself. Expanding our awareness of and deepening our relationship with this life force is called *pranayama*. As we engage in the practice of *pranayama*, the mind becomes enamored with the subtle pulsations of *prana*. The more interested the mind is in the subtle pulsations of *prana*, the steadier it becomes. The roaming tendencies lose their appeal.

Try this simple practice: Watch your breath as it enters and leaves your nostrils. With each inhalation and exhalation notice the quality, texture, coolness or warmth of the breath. Notice the exact place in the nostrils the inhalation touches. Do you experience your thoughts, emotions, and nervous system coming into a more balanced state?

Reflection: This week be with your breath. Reflect on the interconnection between your breath and your inner world and your breath and the outer world. What do you notice?

Limb 5: Pratyahara ~ PULLING IN OF THE SENSES

Pratyahara is a turning. We speak of the turning of the earth from season to season. We speak of the turning of the years, the decades, the centuries. We speak of the turning of events. Turnings have a clear demarcation denoting an ending and the next beginning.

When we engage in *pratyahara,* we turn from the outer world to the one within. We turn from sensory engagement in the outer world to inner perception and witnessing of the events unfolding in the inner world. Ceasing to use the mind to engage with the external world, we now have an opportunity to use the mind to study the mind itself.

This turning happens when we shut off external sensory engagement. We find a quiet spot that is free from sensory temptations. This is important because the mind receives a staggering number of impulses per second from each sensory organ. Imagine the impact and amount of thought processing the mind has to do to engage like this.

When we engage in *pratyahara*, we turn from sensory engagement in the outer world, to inner perception. We now have an opportunity to use the mind to study itself.

And so we turn inward, away from the sheer volume of external sensory input, to the softer, subtler movements of the inner world. Here we may discover a profound subtleness not available to us before. Here we may discover that when the senses are turned inward our energy is conserved. Here we may discover that the mind doesn't need external stimuli to roam; it can roam on its own.

Sense withdrawal, along with the previous four limbs, primes us to face, and eventually free, our minds in the practice of the last three limbs.

Try this simple practice: Find a quiet place and time where you won't be disturbed. Using tools from the first four limbs, make yourself comfortable. Now gently close your eyes, keeping your eyes, eyebrows, and face soft and your lips gently together. Explore what is "inside" of you. What do you notice?

Limbs 6, 7, 8: Dharana, Dhyana, Samadhi ~ MEDITATION

These last three limbs are collectively called *samyana* and refer to both the process and the states we think of as meditation. Known respectively as concentration, meditation, and absorption, they lie at the very heart of yoga. I have chosen to write about them collectively because, when we have prepared well, each of these three limbs flow effortlessly into the next.

Our practice of the first five limbs has prepared the environment for these last three limbs. Now, taking a seated position on the floor or in a chair, we bring our body to stillness with steadiness and comfort. Focusing on the breath, we soften ourselves, opening to a deeper rhythmic flow. Withdrawing our senses from the outer world by closing our eyes, we sit still in the quietest place we can find, preferably a place we continuously devote to this practice.

In this process, our mind is asked to do something very different than it is used to. First, instead of being engaged in the outer world, it is being asked to engage with the inner world. Second, instead of multi-tasking, it is being asked to do one thing. And third, instead of being free to change its object of attention, it is being asked to keep its attention on the same object in one continuous flow.

To engage in this process, we focus on the breath or a sacred word or words (*mantra*). Succeeding in this process even for a few seconds is known as concentration. It might sound something like "breath, breath, breath, oh I forgot to put bananas on my shopping list, breath, breath, I can't believe

Mary said that to me, breath, breath, breath." It is a strange process to be engaged in, but we keep bringing the mind back to the breath, our chosen focus.

Over time, we find that we are staying with our focus for longer periods of time. Concentration has become meditation.

Samadhi, or absorption, means we have become so caught up in the focus of our unwavering attention that the ego self disappears; it has become absorbed in the very thing we are focusing on. For that period of time the ego is no longer separate. But the minute we realize we are absorbed in something, we are no longer absorbed because we have returned to knowing ourselves as a separate entity, telling ourselves about our experience.

We all have had times where we experienced absorption. Perhaps we were mesmerized by a beautiful sunset, and suddenly we weren't there; the only thing that existed was the sunset. Or perhaps we were jogging, or working at our computer, and suddenly we weren't there; the only thing that existed was the process of running or creating. In these instances, we have been absorbed in a unifying experience where we are no longer separate. From a place of unity, the view is different; our narratives seem surprisingly limited; our preferences seem surprisingly naïve.

Returning to the example of training a new puppy, and the process of these last three limbs, let's imagine we have a fenced in back yard where our new puppy has been freely exploring, happily smelling different scents, barking at passersby, and running from corner to corner. But now it is time to bring the puppy inside for kenneling. Now it is contained in one space, probably whimpering, circling the kennel, and complaining about restricted freedom. We have placed a chew toy in the kennel to give the puppy something to do. Eventually it calms down, settles into a restful, curled up position, and stays, contented with the chew toy. And so it is with our minds.

We are continually preparing for meditation through our practice of the *yamas & niyamas*, *asana*, and breath (*pranayama*). With sense withdrawal (*pratyahara*) we have taken the mind out of its freedom to "play outside" with external sensory stimuli and "brought it inside" to focus on the inner world. By focusing the mind at the nostrils (this is but one place we can place our attention), we have "kenneled" the mind. And by asking the mind to focus on the breath as it enters and leaves the nostrils or on a sacred word or words (a *mantra*), we have given the mind a "chew toy," something it can occupy itself with. Now we sit. We listen.

For many of us with tired, over stimulated minds, we may find ourselves complaining, much like a new puppy when it is brought inside and kenneled. I often hear it said, "I can't meditate," or "meditation makes my mind worse." What we are really saying is that for the first time we can see the unruliness of our own mind. This is the bad news, but it is also the good news.

In 2015, a University of Virginia psychology professor,

Timothy Wilson, led a study to test the human capacity to sit still and just be with their minds. He set up an experiment where individuals (of all ages) could sit in a room quietly by themselves for 15 minutes, or self-administer a mild electric shock. The outcome of the study was that 67% of the men and 25% of the women shocked themselves at least once during that time period. They preferred the shock to the silence.

The French philosopher and mystic, Blaise Pascal, made the statement that, "All of humanity's problems stem from our inability to sit quietly in a room alone." Perhaps as we discover what sits in our minds, we can begin to appreciate his statement as well as the results of the University of Virginia study.

Yet it is meditation that frees us from our entanglement in the *kleshas*. Yoga Sutra chapter 2, verse 11 tells us that the roaming tendencies can be destroyed in meditation. It is in these still moments on our cushion or chair that we are practicing the ability to sit in whatever arises (appealing or revolting) and not react to it. We are learning to avoid oscillating between clinging and resisting. In the process, our minds are being purified and stabilized from their wandering habits. The slow, steady power of this process is easy to underestimate.

My Octopus Teacher is a 2020 Netflix documentary about Craig Foster and the year he spent embarking on a relationship with an octopus. Prior to this year, Craig was feeling burned out and searching for a deeper meaning to his life. In 2010, he decided to spend a year diving in an underwater kelp forest near Cape Town, South Africa.

His habit was to dive daily into these waters, filming what he encountered. Although the water was quite chilly, he chose to dive without a wetsuit, allowing himself to be more vulnerable and receptive to whatever he came across. He ended up encountering an octopus and over time, befriending it. As trust and intimacy were gained, Craig Foster's life was forever changed.

Most of us don't have the opportunity for an experience like Craig's, and yet we do. Meditation offers us a yet unknown, unexplored region that we can return to daily. And like Craig, we can choose to go there vulnerable and receptive. Trust and intimacy can be built up over the daily encounters we have there. And our life can be forever changed.

> There is a sweetness the mind enjoys as the power to flow peacefully becomes more interesting than wandering to and fro. Equanimity is becoming a more permanent way of feeling and being.

There is a sweetness the mind enjoys as the power to flow peacefully becomes more interesting than wandering to and fro. Before a diet of practice and nonattachment, the mind didn't want to come indoors; it wanted to keep playing outside. But now it relishes its peaceful time; in fact, the growing experience of wellbeing it feels is beginning to be sustained in other activities.

Equanimity is becoming a more permanent way of feeling and being.

When my children were young, we often cleared off the table, covered it with blankets draped to the floor, and created a dark, closed-in space under the table. No longer a place we sat to eat, this piece of furniture had been transformed into a "fort." My children entered with anticipation, wide-eyed and quiet. They sensed there was something special about that dark, closed-in space. They didn't know what it was; but they loved being there. Except for an occasional giggle or whisper, they were happy to just sit there quietly, oblivious to all their toys, which remained outside their fort.

Over time, our minds themselves are transformed into an inner fort of wonder and equanimity where we can hang out whether we are sitting quietly in meditation or fully engaged in a busy day.

Try this simple practice: Take a position on the floor or in a chair where you can be still. Bring yourself into a harmonious feeling through appreciation, gratitude, or prayer. Find your still place of steadiness and comfort. Make sure your head, neck, and trunk are in a straight line. Close your eyes gently, soften your face, and watch your breath at the nostrils. When your mind wanders, gently bring it back to the breath at the nostrils. Stay here as long as you are able.

Reflection: This week ponder the words of Blaise Pascal that "All of humanity's problems stem from our inability to sit quietly in a room alone." Do you agree? Why or why not?

Vairagya ~ NONATTACHMENT (PARTNER OF PRACTICE)

One of my friends has been practicing yoga for many years. At first, her practice was irregular, on again off again. But one day something changed. Her practice became the most important thing in her life, and she made a firm commitment to practice daily without fail, a commitment she has remained faithful to.

On her journey to becoming the best practitioner she could be, she decided that she needed to deal with what she called her addiction to dark chocolate. This went on for months. She would quit for a while and then start again, only to become more frustrated and more determined. I listened as this process unfolded, which mostly entailed periodically throwing out the chocolate she had in the house, only to buy more chocolate a few days later while at the store.

One day she called me and announced triumphantly that she had come up with a winning plan. She had placed all the chocolate she could find in her house into her safe deposit box, locked it securely, and then taken the key to the neighbor. She was confident in this new plan of hers. Because the neighbor held the key to her safe box, she was sure she could go on with her life, victorious over the chocolate. As you can imagine, it didn't take too many days before she went back to her neighbor, asking for the key.

My friend's relationship with dark chocolate not only delights me with its humorous unfolding, it also epitomizes what many of us do when we try to make a change. We go to war with habits we don't want, and we usually lose. We deny them only to notice they have returned with reinforcements. We make resolutions and promises that in no time are broken. None of our strategies work; in fact they seem to give more power to the very thing we were hoping to rid ourselves of, leaving us little energy to focus on the things we do want.

Looking at the example of my friend through the eyes of Patanjali, we see her strategy was in error. Not only was she fighting what she didn't want, it was consuming much of her thought process. She kept coming up with new ways to win the next battle, but was losing the war. Like many of us who use this strategy, she was frustrated, self-critical, and tired of defeat.

What we fight, fix, fear, blame, deny, or suppress only gets stronger.

What we fight, fix, fear, blame, deny, or suppress only gets stronger. My friend was trying to control her desire for dark chocolate by fighting it; this way of thinking was not bringing any peace to her mind. I'm reminded of Pandit Rajmani Tigunait's insight that trying to have a peaceful mind by using unpeaceful methods does not bring peace. For change to happen, we need to turn our minds towards higher virtues like compassion, and keep the mind in a steady, peaceful flow.

This all sounds great. But we have spent our entire lives heavily investing in the *kleshas*. We have created strong neural pathways for comforting ourselves with our favorite versions of excess and poor me stories. We have created strong neural pathways that leap to judgment of others and to

144

simmering in self-righteous anger when we feel slighted. We have created a mind that is bored with too much quiet and simplicity. These things live in our tissues and nervous system; they feel real; they are the world we know.

How do we reconcile this lived visceral experience with the seemingly simply recommendation to "chill" and let these things go? What does it even mean to be nonattached? Nonattachment is not some pie-in-the-sky-feely-good pretending that nothing is bothering us. It is not denial; it is not suppression; it is not spiritual bypassing. (Spiritual bypassing is the practice of pretending to be spiritual without doing the hard work involved. It was first noticed by John Welwood in the 1980's and expanded in a book by Robert Augustus Masters.) It does not equate to indifference, compliance, passivity, or non-action. It does not involve lying to ourselves. Nonattachment first involves a willingness to be aware.

An awareness practice:

Be aware that you carry an image of the world, yourself, and how things should and shouldn't be with you everywhere you go. Be aware that every situation is you imposing your story on the moment. Every ripple of tension in your body is embedded in this story of yours. Every emotional reaction is linked to this story. Nonattachment begins with the courageous act of acknowledging these facts and seeing how they get played out in life.

Learn to feel how clinging and resisting feel inside you. Do you tighten your jaw or maybe your shoulders? Does your breath become shallow or held? Do you feel angry, self-righteous, judgmental, excited? How do these things find expression in you? What is the narrative you habitually associate with them?

Sit with the disturbance long enough to identify it. Be willing to notice the tension in your body.....and then be willing to soften into it. Be willing to notice the intensity of emotion..... and then be willing to sit in the emotion until it passes. Be willing to notice the narrative you are telling yourself about what is happening.....and then be willing to let go of the story/concepts and sit with what is present when you keep narrative at bay.

Here is the real opportunity. This is the work. This is where the disturbance is, where the clinging and resisting lie, where we grip life, where our selfish impulses live. Everything that pulls our mind to other than its innate peaceful flow shows us what is in our way. We don't have to go looking for our attachments, they freely present themselves to us. We have taken a lifetime to create them, and they are readily available to us. The question is, are we available to see them, soften into them, learn from them, and then let them go? "Perfection is achieved not when there is nothing left to add," says Antoine de Saint-Exupéry, "but when there is nothing left to take away."

> Are we available to see our attachments, soften into them, learn from them, and then let them go?

Buddha was able to see through attachments. When he sat under the bodhi tree, he was able to see that sure, what was tempting him would be pleasurable for a while, but after that....well, not so much so. He was able to see that indulgence, whether in fleshly pleasures, anger, or greed, all eventually had an unpleasant ending. He didn't grab onto his attachments or avoid his repulsions; he saw through them. He didn't fight for his preferences, he saw the full trajectory of their illusion and eventual disappointment. And so he continued to sit there. He wanted to know what was there when the *kleshas* weren't.

It's not that sensory pleasure or having preferences is a bad thing. After all, the world (and that includes our bodies) is meant to be enjoyed. It's simply that from a place of bondage, our misplaced desires often drive us to act without thinking, almost always resulting in harm to others or ourselves. As our awareness of and softening into our attachments grow, we are freer to enjoy sensory pleasure sensibly. We are able to enjoy without causing harm. This is a huge contribution to ourselves, our communities, and ultimately to world peace.

Nonattachment, also translated as dispassion, is a word my spouse and I get tangled up in when we discuss its meaning. He doesn't like the word. To him it sounds like not caring; it's too distancing and apathetic sounding. He feels as human beings we are called to care and be caring, to act in this world and make it a better place. I couldn't agree with him more. So maybe the real question is, how does nonattachment, caring, and action/inaction all go together?

An awareness practice:

Have you ever spoken words to someone that you would do anything to take back? I know I have, more than once. We get somehow thrown off balance because a person is not acting "the way they should." And before we can stop ourselves, the words have come out, strung together in what later becomes an embarrassing moment for us. Or what about the times you didn't act or say something that later you'd give anything to go back in time and say because the words you didn't say were not only appropriate but necessary.

Have you ever felt immobilized by the immensity of the challenges facing your family, your country, or the world? So immobilized that you knew you had to do something, but you didn't know what that something was? The caring is real; there is just a huge chasm between the caring and the ability to know how to respond.

Reflect on a particular incident when your response was inappropriate for the situation. Perhaps you responded hastily and harshly. Perhaps you didn't respond at all. Can you correlate the visceral feeling of your inappropriate response with a particular belief? Did you feel powerful or powerless in your response?

We live with many inappropriate actions and inactions because what lies between us and right action is a sea of conditioning. When we can only see our story of how things should be and then impose that story on the situation, our response falls short of impeccability. Real caring and appropriate action happen in proportion to our ability to see the conditioning we are bringing to the situation. The more we can see our conditioning in the moment, the more we can respond appropriately with genuine care.

My biggest learning as a yoga teacher came early. I was freshly out of my intensive teacher training with Yogi Bhajan and a nervous, excited new teacher. Sitting stately on my sheepskin, dressed entirely in white, I waited as the room filled. As class progressed, the energy was palpable. I felt satisfied and full. But all was not as I had thought.

A regular student had brought a friend with her who was suffering from depression and a series of challenges in her life. The friend never returned to the studio; she had experienced the class as too "happy." I was too smiley; my class was too upbeat. My need to have everyone feel good during class interfered with this friend's ability to find a place that felt safe to her. I had to learn to create space where students could come and be who they are, where the practice could work in them in ways I was not privy to, and where my role was as a conduit not a cheerleader. I needed to learn to be nonattached to everyone feeling good in my class. It was also necessary to become aware that my needing others to be different than they were, created a form of violence on their right to feel what they were feeling.

Our subtle and not so subtle attempts to cling to or resist anything in our environment or in ourselves is one of the ways we find ourselves stuck in the bondage of attachment. Any attempt to make something the way we think it should be, including a yoga class or our own practice, thwarts the grace that wants to find us.

This is true whatever our role. Can we allow ourselves to be who we are in this moment? Can we allow ourselves to have the feeling we have in this moment? Can we sit as a student at the feet of life and allow life to be what it is? Can we discern correct action while remaining nonattached?

When Mataji (Narvada Puri) spoke on this subject, she said, "Everyday life gives you an opportunity to test your equanimity." It was clear she placed a high value on the equanimity that comes with nonattachment, so it wasn't surprising when she went on to say that we had to "give up a little of our happiness to give up our sadness," and that a good practice for nonattachment was to "need less, not more."

I have had many years to ponder her words and still they seem wiser than I am able to comprehend, but the implications are clear.

Clinging and resisting are opposite sides of the same process; if we are free from one, we gain freedom from the other. The more freedom we gain from both, the more equanimity we have. Imagine what it must be like to live in the roller coaster life presents us and not be pulled off center. In these moments of some form of victory over our attachments, there is a sense of freedom and satisfaction. These moments feel spacious and calm; there is more of us present.

150

Sitting at my father's bedside in the hospital, I wondered if he would survive this particular stay. Alone with him, I asked, "Dad, how do you feel about dying?" He smiled and looked at me with tender eyes as he responded, "Well if I die, I get to be with Jesus; if I live, I get to stay here with Nancy [his wife]. Either way, I win." He died a week later having said prayers of gratitude for the experience of his life and crying as he embraced Nancy. With honesty and nonattachment, he died peacefully.

What stands between us and our higher selves is our attachments. Some have a strong hold on us, others not so much. Some have been with us our entire lives; others are more recent additions. Sometimes we need to let go. Sometimes we need to act. Sometimes we just need to sit in the grief we are feeling and mourn whatever we have lost.

My brother Doug and his wife lost their cabin and 40 acres of land to one of Colorado's wildfires. They were devastated. My brother found relevance in the Biblical story of Jonah, who was swallowed by a big fish and spent three days in the belly of the fish singing praises. By taking solace in the story of Jonah, my brother faced his loss by grieving and giving gratitude.

I often wonder what my dad and brother did in the years preceding these events that allowed them to meet loss with such grace. In an incident in my life, I was not so graceful.

151

I was reeling from the sting of betrayal from someone I loved dearly. The event continued to play in my mind and heart. I could feel bitterness and sadness overtaking me, and I couldn't find a way to shake it. Much later I had the opportunity to sit with Swami Avdheshanand Giri and ask him for help. Feeling the heaviness of my heart, I asked him, "How do you have a pure heart?" He smiled at me with such love and said, "Give it all to God; just keep giving it to God."

I didn't know what that meant exactly, so I started experimenting. When the story was in my head and the heaviness was in my heart (which was quite often in the beginning) I attempted to give it over to something else. I didn't know how, so I silently said things like, "God, I don't know how to do this, but my heart is heavy; please take this." I had tried and failed on my own; now I surrendered it as best I could. In time, my heart began to mend and feel light again, and the story I had been telling myself began to loosen its grip on my mind.

What I didn't realize at the time was that I had made an enemy of feeling betrayed and then "gone to war" with it to try to stop it. I didn't want to feel that way so I tried to stop feeling that way. The act of trying to "push away" that feeling had in a subtle way attached me to it. I was seeking to have a peaceful mind, but I was doing it with unpeaceful methods. I was fighting what I didn't want. When I was able to accept the feelings and then surrender them (note that both acceptance and surrender are peaceful methods), I began to heal.

In whatever way we meet the difficulties in our life, it is important to peacefully digest these painful experiences so they can be integrated in the present and not leave us stuck in the past. Nonattachment is not gripping, but it is not ignoring either. It is a replacement of our pettiness and irritation as well as a full digestion of our wounds, trauma, and significant losses.

Acknowledgment of our tendencies, of what the body clings to and what it fights, is important. We need to know ourselves otherwise we continue to repeat ourselves in oblivious ignorance. But it is equally important that we don't waste time wallowing in negative self-judgment and regrets. Our attachments are already taking too much of our energy; why give them more and bruise ourselves in the process? As one of my friends so bluntly put it, "Once I've identified it as vomit, why would I want to pick it up and eat it?"

If we really understood the value of seeing ourselves in action, we would be grateful because now we know what stands between us and our higher way of being. Our focus and energy would automatically go to creating a practice stronger

153

than our weakness. As Dr. David Frawley reminds us, "Inner peace must become our dominant force. We should no longer seek to overcome our pain but to develop our joy" (Frawley, p. 42).

Reflection: Notice the times your mind keeps coming back to an attachment. A friend describes this as similar to a tongue that keeps coming back to a bad tooth. How would you describe this process of being attached? What are you getting out of "feeling this bad tooth"?

Reflection: Name something that is holding you captive to the past because you haven't digested or integrated it. What does this "something" need? Is it to be grieved, forgiven, ritualized, supported by a therapist, or....? What in you is asking to be healed?

Reflection: Can you let the past, the present, others, and yourself be as they are and still work for change and a desired future reality? How do we reconcile acceptance of what is with our hopes and dreams of a better "us" and a better world in the future?

Between Stimulus & Response

Viktor Frankl was an Austrian neurologist and psychiatrist. I read his book *Man's Search for Meaning* at an impressionable young age and was overcome by his experiences as a prisoner in Nazi concentration camps. Under dire circumstances, he discovered he had the power to choose his response to the horror happening around him. At the time, I was taken aback by this bold proclamation of the power of choice.

Frankl was speaking to the gap between what is happening around us and what we choose to do with it, referred to as the space between stimulus and response. He recognized that whatever the circumstances, this was the space of choice; this was the place of human autonomy. My entire training in somatic education was based on consciously focusing on this space to bring about change in unconscious habitual patterns.

There is a choice point between the sensory input and what we choose to do with it. Within this space is the opportune moment to practice inner freedom. This is the space within which Viktor Frankl, under the most horrendous conditions, redirected his mind and became the master of his life. Years later, Nelson Mandela was to realize the same reality. As a prisoner on Robben Island, he held words from *Invictus* by

> The only real freedom any of us have is the choice of how we will respond (vs. react) to the outer world and how we will deal with our conditioning.

the poet William Ernest Henley, close to his heart. The words "I am the master of my fate; I am the captain of my soul," produced a man of character and compassion in the harshest of environments.

The only real freedom any of us have is the choice of how we will respond (vs. react) to the outer world and how we will deal with our conditioning. We could illustrate this understanding like this:

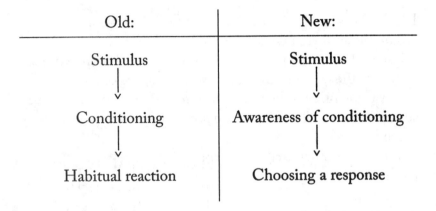

Old:	New:
Stimulus	Stimulus
↓	↓
Conditioning	Awareness of conditioning
↓	↓
Habitual reaction	Choosing a response

In the first scenario, the impulse comes to us (either from the outside or the inside), we quickly and unconsciously run it through our conditioning, and we react in accordance with our conditioning. It's a fast reaction and happens by default.

In the second scenario, something comes to us, and we take advantage of the space created by witnessing our thoughts to respond in a choiceful way. Awareness gives us the chance to recalculate our response if need be. This is not a war on our mind but a redirection of energy. It is the ability to bounce back, recover, catch ourselves, and change course.

Even at age four, my granddaughter Lucy understood that she had the ability to watch her mind and have some autonomy over her choices. In one conversation she told me, "Grandma, sometimes my brain talks to me." I said, "What does it say?" She responded, "It tells me to do mean things." I said, "What do you do then?" She replied, "I tell my brain that would be mean, so I'm not going to do it."

Seeing what we are thinking and/or doing puts our conditioning out in front of our face, so to speak. Once it is out in the open, it suddenly takes its place among other possible choices. Now we see that this isn't **the** way, but one of many possibilities. Awareness creates choice, and choice creates freedom.

We don't have to fight ourselves or fix ourselves. We just get to see; and then we get to choose. Each time we choose a more thoughtful response, our conditioned reaction begins to lose its power over us.

We don't have to fight ourselves or our habits. We don't have to fix or change ourselves. We just get to see; we get to know ourselves and our tendencies along with the narrative that runs us. And then we get to choose. Each time we choose a more thoughtful response, our conditioned reaction begins to lose its power over us.

This does not mean we have found a place devoid of inner and outer turmoil. Regrets, grief, sadness, disappointment, and more, move through our inner world as surely as storms move through our outer world. We just get better at being stable with the changes of weather. It is not a weakness to see our attachments and resistance; if these are the cause of our bondage, then it seems like a gift to see the things that stand between ourselves and our freedom.

> It is not a weakness to see our attachments and resistance; if these are the cause of our bondage, then it seems like a gift to see the things that stand between ourselves and our freedom.

Every experience gives us a chance to be entangled or not. What we learn in our sitting meditation, we take into daily life. We learn to slow down, to pay attention, to choose how we will respond. If we get entangled, we suffer, but we also learn. Our small failings during the day are a reminder of the cost of entanglement to ourselves and others. We take responsibility for being the cause and source of our own inner turmoil.

"Pause" is a word that has made its way into mainline vernacular as a reminder to think before we act. From behavioral psychologists, to neurologists, to spiritual teachers, we hear words of caution to pause for a moment. This reflective pause can prevent us from doing something that might later prove regrettable. This reflective pause is the crucial opportunity between stimulus and response.

The question always before us is, are we serving our self-centeredness or our generosity? Our anxiety or our trust? Our disturbance or our contentment? It is in these everyday choices between stimulus and response, that we deepen our bondage to the *kleshas* or our freedom from them.

An awareness exercise: Take the Harvard Implicit Bias Test (https://implicit.harvard.edu). You will find a variety of subjects to test yourself on. Discover if your unconscious mind believes differently than your conscious mind. How do your answers reflect the power of the narratives that have shaped you?

Reflection: When you make a choiceful response between stimulus and response, what guides your choice, i.e., what influences your response? Are you focused on the outcome, a personal need, an ethical guideline, or....?

Reflection: This week practice being the "captain" of your choices.

Your Mind on Practice & Nonattachment

The first bridge over Niagara Falls was built in 1855, spanned 800 feet, and connected Niagara Falls, Ontario and Niagara Falls, New York. The vision for such a bridge belonged to Canadian politician William Hamilton Merritt, but the implementation of such a vision was met with skepticism among engineers. John Augustus Roebling was one of only four who submitted plans for such a bridge and was eventually awarded the contract.

Now Roebling faced the difficult problem of how to get an initial line of contact over the turbulent waters to connect the Canadian side with the United States side. After many brainstorming sessions with his men, Roebling settled on the idea of a kite flying contest with a prize to the boy who could fly his kite in such a way that it would land on the other side. The prize went to 16-year-old Homan Walsh who was able to accomplish such a feat and land his kite so that it secured a thin string attaching Canadian soil with American soil.

Once the engineers had the line of connection, they could now draw larger and stronger lines across the kite string, eventually running a ⅞ inch cable that, when the bridge reached completion, held pedestrians, carriages, and trains.

The mind on a diet of practice and nonattachment is similar to this process. Our unruly minds are hard to navigate in the turbulent waters of life. But practice and nonattachment, like that initial kite string, make possible a foundation that over time becomes stronger and steadier. The turbulence below does not go away; we just get better at maneuvering it while staying in equanimity. Our minds can bear the heavy traffic of life with clarity and tranquility.

But all of this takes time. Our conditioning, habits, and tendencies have various degrees of strength (Yoga Sutra 2:4). Like weeds in a garden, some can be easily pulled up, others have deeper root systems and are more difficult to deal with. Like an intact, underground root system, the tendency to roam is still a plausible pathway. Even when things seem calm, vigilance is needed.

What is happening in this process? Technically, the roaming tendencies of the mind are being replaced by meditative tendencies, which act to restrain roaming. And unlike the roaming tendencies which disturb the mind, meditative tendencies bring peace, joy, and inner contentment to the mind. The mind is gradually being changed.

Do we become better people in this process? I don't know. Some days I would say yes, other days I would answer no. Until the *kleshas* are destroyed in the deeper recesses of meditation and the roaming tendencies are

On a diet of practice and nonattachment, the mind gets clearer. We start making choices for a sustained contentment rather than choices that keep us on a pleasure/pain roller coaster.

161

mastered, we will get triggered. However, it is the steady diet of practice and nonattachment that allows us to acknowledge and regulate ourselves when we are triggered and offers us the freedom to choose our response.

On a diet of practice and nonattachment, the mind gets clearer. It's as if we have been living in a dark tunnel, and now we are standing on top of a mountain. The view has changed. We are able to see the magnitude and depth of the obstacles in our way and the demons that haunt us. We "catch" ourselves more frequently and more quickly. This may not seem like much, but it is enormous. It gives us the growing power of self understanding, along with the power of choice. Because we are able to see the far-reaching consequences of satisfying an immediate impulse, we pause to consider the value of such a choice. We start making choices for a sustained contentment rather than choices that keep us on a pleasure/pain roller coaster.

This growing clarity is called *viveka,* or the power of discernment. Discernment allows us to see how self-defeating it has been to burden the outside world with our expectations and neediness. And in some strange way, that realization allows us to more fully enjoy the people and things around us. We come to know there is nothing we can do to make an experience last, and in that knowing, experience becomes more vibrant.

Discernment allows us to realize how connected we are to all things. Thinking only about our own wellbeing no longer makes sense. We realize that a war or a drought on the other side of the planet affects us. Injustice, oppression, inequality, lies, corruption affect us. This awareness prompts us to action, guided by wisdom and fueled by compassion.

Together, practice and nonattachment create the quiet space where awareness can flourish.

Together, practice and nonattachment create the quiet space where awareness can flourish.

More subtle components enter our reality, and we begin to see that we are guilty of the things we blame others for. We become aware of the intelligence of our own bodies and learn to listen to them. We learn the language that spirit speaks and heed its guidance. Life becomes more fulfilling in this body, on this earth. The mind is becoming our friend.

Reflection: How do you understand practice and nonattachment working together in your life?

Reflection: How is your practice (or how might your practice be) similar to the first bridge built over Niagara Falls? Does it feel more like a kite string or a cable? Can you identify with the turbulent waters under the bridge? How might this imagery sustain your daily attention to practice and nonattachment?

Obstacles

Mahatma Gandhi was a lover of truth, and because he was a lover of truth, India was freed from British rule. Because he was a lover of truth, the world recognized and respected him. Because he was a lover of truth, Gandhi consistently sought after and experimented with truth in his own life.

In Yoga Sutra 1:30 & 31, Patanjali, I think, is inviting us to be a lover of truth concerning ourselves and the lived reality of our habits and tendencies. In these verses he gives a list of what this lived reality might look like. In verse 30, he states, "Disease, mental inertia, doubt, carelessness, sloth, inability to withdraw from sense cravings, clinging to misunderstanding, inability to reach the goal [*samadhi*], and inability to retain it throw our mind outward; they are obstacles" (Tigunait, p. 144). As if this wasn't enough, he follows with five more in verse 31: "Pain, mental agitation, unsteadiness or trembling of limbs, [abnormal or disturbed] inhalation and [abnormal or disturbed] exhalation all arise with the obstacles" (Tigunait, p. 151).

These two verses lay out a vivid account of the cost of our bondage to the *kleshas*, and the words are not sugar coated. A result of our roaming tendencies, this cascade of afflictions builds one on top of the other taking us deeper and deeper into dis-ease. If Patanjali was writing today, he might use words like stress, high blood pressure, anxiety, inflammation, leaky gut, trouble sleeping, frazzled, unmotivated, lack of confidence, and feelings of despair and hopelessness.

These obstacles (also referred to as disturbances) are both the result of our entanglement in the *kleshas* and obstacles to our unentanglement. As such, they are both humbling and informative. First, they allow us to honestly assess the current damage the *kleshas* have done in our own lives. This assessment gives us a starting place. Second, they allow us to understand and shape our practice in an effective way. This helps us stay focused on our own needs and not compare our practice to someone else. And third, the obstacles inspire our commitment and dedication to our practice. Without this honest assessment, it is too easy to make excuses, blame others, and lack a sense of direction. Love of the truth allows us to face these obstacles with clarity and commitment.

It takes courage to look truthfully at the list above and recognize that every time the *kleshas* hijack our minds, they drain our energy, rattle our nervous system, and cloud our awareness. It takes courage to look truthfully at the list above and find our current place on that list. But if we are willing to tell ourselves the truth, our practice can become a powerful tool.

> It takes courage to recognize that every time the *kleshas* hijack our minds, they drain our energy, rattle our nervous system, and cloud our awareness.

A few years ago, I was sitting in an auditorium with other students listening to Pandit Rajmani Tigunait lecture when he spoke to the importance of looking at the obstacles that get in our way. He talked about how easy it is for us to get caught trying to put together the perfect practice or to strive for the goals that will improve our life. Then he suggested that we look closely at the big stuff in our way, and make facing that stuff an integral part of the practice.

In that moment, I recognized myself in his words. I was aware of the amount of time I often spend skillfully planning my practice. I was also aware of the amount of things I shove aside because I don't "have time" to deal with them. I wasn't facing my obstacles.

For the past decade my spouse and I had gotten too busy to attend well to all the pieces of our lives. The basement became the place that held the expanding clutter of our increasing imbalance. Things began to pile up. We could hardly move around, but we conveniently kept ignoring the truth of the situation because the rest of the house was pleasantly tidy.

Besides, my sights were set on accomplishing things that "had value" and toward growing myself through my practice, not on being a basement cleaner. But heeding Pandit Rajmani Tigunait's words, I swallowed my pride and grandiose ideas, went to the basement, and began the arduous task before me.

This is a hard story for me to share, both because it is a glaring first world problem, and also because it is so unglamorous. What I wish I could convey is the incredible gifts that came from facing this biggest obstacle in my life at that time. In many ways it was a reckoning with shadow parts of me, it was a reminder of the incredible gifts and joys in my life, and it was a stark call to balance. The whole process purified the air (inside and outside of me) and it created space (inside and outside of me). I could breathe more freely in my home; I could breathe more freely in my body.

Not all obstacles have to do with cleaning basements. Sometimes the biggest obstacle confronting us is our inability to forgive (ourselves or someone else), or our inability to leave social media once we sign in, or our inability to resist food that holds no nutritional value for us, or our need to hold another in a possessive grip.

The obstacles are a burden. They hinder our ability to focus, to think kind thoughts, to sit still, and to be quiet. The valuable lesson I learned from my basement experience was to take a truthful look at these obstacles and then to make addressing them a continuous part of my practice.

> It takes a great deal of energy to hide things from ourselves. True practice includes facing those things in us that need facing.

It takes a great deal of energy to hide things from ourselves. Not facing obstacles drains our precious vitality. Brianna Wiest made an insightful observation about selfcare when she said, "True self-care is not salt baths and chocolate cake, it is making the choice to build a life you don't need to regularly escape from." I would use her words to echo that true practice includes facing those things in us that need facing.

With deaths from suicide, alcoholism, and drug addiction

rising in the United States, one has to wonder what is really going on in a country that portrays itself as the land of freedom and opportunity for all. What truths are we individually and collectively unwilling to see and deal with? These are hard realities that are much easier to ignore, but we do so at our own peril.

Our egos often seek impressive images and practices where we can entertain self-aggrandizing thoughts about ourselves, but the obstacles often send us to the shadow work in the basement of our lives. This process requires humility and a willingness to face the truth of our lives.

Reflection: What is your biggest obstacle? How is this obstacle taking your energy? In what way(s) is this obstacle interfering with your practice? Why are you avoiding it? What do you need to do to attend to this obstacle so that it is no longer a burden?

Reflection: Do you agree that facing our obstacles requires humility and a willingness to face the truth of our lives? Why or why not?

Daily Life ~ *EVEN A LITTLE EFFORT*

During a class session many years ago, I was given a handout by Yogiraj Achala that stated in big bold letters: *Pardon the Mess; Transformation in Process*. We students chuckled and then dutifully put the handout in our binder along with our notes. As I sit in the seeming chaos of the global pandemic and all its repercussions, I see the truth of these words. The question is, do I see the truth of this process in my own life?

The great teachers tell us there is something major that wants to happen to us; we are blueprinted to be transformed. Not the ego's idea of transformation, but a transformation that is beyond our current understanding. This is why so often it seems we are regressing, not progressing, as we

From the view of the ego, things are not moving along as planned or hoped for. But from the soul's perspective, the process is perfect.

engage in our yoga practice. From the view of the ego, things are not moving along as planned or hoped for. But from the soul's perspective, the process is perfect.

In a life that is constantly changing and a mind that changes with it, we are slowly building stability and equanimity. This is a tall order.

A caterpillar has to disintegrate into a soupy mess in order to emerge with the ability to fly. As a caterpillar, it could only crawl; now, as a butterfly, it can soar. The caterpillar that fights this process or tries to make it happen never gets to fly. Likewise, when we fight this process in us or try to make it happen on our terms, we damage our own process.

We hurt ourselves when we think things should be other than they are; that we should be other than we are, or that the process of our transformation should look different than it does. As we learn to surrender and trust, we begin to willingly enter the cocoon and submit to becoming the soupy mess of someone in the process of being transformed. This is good news, even though it may look messy.

But on one particularly messy day, I forgot all of this. I wallowed for a time in self-denigration because I wasn't doing enough. I wasn't doing enough practice, or enough for my family and friends, or enough to stop world hunger and planetary devastation. I was a terrible person in just about every way I could think of.

Out of my despondency, I realized if I just spent 51% of my day consciously training my mind, I would be moving towards freedom and away from entanglement. I couldn't help but laugh as I thought: Deborah Adele's 51% plan ~ the scenic route to enlightenment.

It was my way of acknowledging that being hard on myself was not at all helpful. I remembered hearing Pandit Rajmani Tigunait say that "the first recipient of our negative thoughts is ourselves." I was experiencing the weight of my own negativity towards myself twofold. And this was not the kind of mind I wanted to live in.

I don't know what my unique process looks like any more than I know what being free of the *kleshas* looks like. My ego, under its current misperception, has no way of understanding these things. I also can't compare my process to anyone else; the cocoon I spin will be a little different.

People have different ways of getting their bodies into a cold lake. Some like to jump right in and feel it all at once; others take it slow, beginning with their big toe and methodically, inch-by-inch, invite the rest to follow. Some days just seem like the latter. Much of life is a combination of the two.

In the revered text, the Bhagavad Gita, Krishna leads the despondent Arjuna on a path from bondage to victory. The text is rich with wisdom

> Our effort never goes to waste, and there is no failure.

and guidance and foreshadows Patanjali's writing in the Yoga Sutra. One verse is particularly comforting. In chapter 2, verse 40 Krishna tells Arjuna that our effort never goes to waste, and there is no failure.

It's valuable to remember these words, especially on days we ourselves may be feeling despondent. The mind field is subtly changed every time we "bring it back." The powers of attention and tranquility are increased, and the power of the roaming tendencies is decreased. Effort is never wasted.

When my spouse and I chose to buy a home, we settled on an older home, knowing that inevitably repairs would need to happen, especially in the bathroom. As things worsened, we could no longer deny that our bathroom had to be totally gutted. Water could barely trickle through the old plumbing. Mold, in spite of our attempts, continued to peek through the ceiling and spread at will. The crack in the bottom of the bathtub threatened to break through at an inopportune time. There was nothing salvageable. We had to do something drastic; the bathroom had to be totally gutted and re-made.

I am struck with the parallels to our minds. If we are honest, we will admit that resentments, worry, and negativity clog the channels of our mind so clarity and grace have trouble flowing through. Greed, jealousy, anger, and fear creep through our fervent attempts to be people of character and courage. Cracks in our thinking lead to poor choices and hurtful actions. At some point we can no longer deny that our minds are in need of some drastic remodeling.

Training our mind is a kinder process than gutting a bathroom, although it may not seem that way at times. There are always surprises, unforeseen challenges, and delays that make it seem like the project will never be complete. Will my bathroom ever be done? Will my mind ever be stable? Will I always live in that uncomfortable place between chaos and promise?

There was another piece to gutting our bathroom. All the piping had to be replaced. The old rusted piping was taken out and new piping was put in its place. When the bathroom was complete, none of the new piping showed. Although it was actually quite beautiful, it wasn't visible. But when we turned on the water, the new pipes allowed for a clear, full water flow. The completed bathroom was lovely, but the real functionality came from the inner gutting that replaced old pipes with new pipes.

The process of training our minds is similar. The work is interior, where no one can see. It is not only important what we do, but how we do it. What is the inner piping of our minds and hearts? Who are we when no one is looking? What is going on behind the scenes of our actions?

The documentary entitled *The Way I See It* is about Pete Souza, the Chief Official White House photographer during the Reagan and Obama presidencies. Because Souza was allowed such intimate, unstaged time with then President Obama, he was able to capture the character of President Obama in several different scenarios such as playing with his children, his relationship with his wife, Michelle, and his exchanges with the staff as well as world leaders.

The result of Souza's photography is the portrayal in pictures of what this man's character looked like behind the scenes. I couldn't help but wonder if someone followed me around with a camera in every situation of my life, what would the still life photos reveal about my character?

Most of us are householders with varying degrees of responsibility. We have bills to pay, family members to care for, relationships to tend, laundry to do, cooking and dishes and cleaning, income to bring in, and unforeseen challenges to meet. Life is not easy. But the one thing we all have is the ability to tend our minds, no matter what our circumstance.

Whether we are on our cushion, or mat, or tending to our daily responsibilities, can we be vigilant to the inner work?

While watching *Won't You Be My Neighbor?*, a documentary about Fred Rogers, I found myself moved by the gentleness and honesty portrayed by Mr. Rogers towards children. One comment that particularly stayed with me was his invitation to "make goodness attractive."

> Whether we are on our cushion, or mat, or tending to our daily responsibilities, can we be vigilant to the inner work?

In contrast, I was aware of an October 3, 2018 article written by Adam Serwer, a political staff writer for *The Atlantic*. Entitled "The Cruelty is the Point," Serwer suggests that for many in this country, finding pleasure in the suffering of people they hate and fear has become a bonding mechanism that fills the vacancy of cultural loneliness.

We humans are a strange combination of selfish and generous, grandiose and humble, fearful and courageous; we hold the full range of possibilities within us. Often called our lower nature and our higher nature, we only fool ourselves and become dangerous to society if we think we are somehow immune from the tendencies of our lower nature.

It's a choice point for all of us. We can spend our time in default mode, entangled in our conditioning, or we can spend our time attentive to training the mind. In this moment we can choose extremism or reconciliation. In this moment we can choose blame or self-responsibility. In this moment we can choose to fight for our ideology or examine it. In this moment we can cultivate minds of disturbance or minds of peace.

We can attend to the inner landscape. Like the pipes in my remodeled bathroom that are never seen, what comes out will be a much purer quality.

Reflection: Observe yourself this week. Are you looking in the mirror at how you look, or are you looking in your heart for how you love? Are you paying attention to what you have or to what you can share?

Reflection: If someone followed you around with a camera and captured the "behind the scenes" of your life, what would the photos reveal about your character, integrity, and empathy?

Questioning the Narrative

My father's childhood was deeply impacted by the depression. He carried the memory of going to bed night after night with gnawing hunger pains that made it difficult to sleep. He carried the memory of wearing old hand-me-downs that were either so big he tripped on the pant legs or so small they constricted his movement. He also carried the memory of watching his own jovial, generous father sink into a deep mental depression when his once flourishing business failed. It was a depression his father never recovered from. Determined to protect we three children from a similar experience, my father set out to live the American dream. And he succeeded.

I am told that money for baby food was scarce when I, the first born, arrived. But by the time I was old enough to recall my growing up years, it was anything but scarce. Our homes were getting bigger and newer and so were our cars. There were plenty of homemade meals on the table (thanks, Mom) and there were yearly family trips to faraway places. There was the opportunity of a good education and the elation of an occasional frilly dress.

Except for the normal year-by-year figuring out what it means to grow up, my only disgruntlement was watching doors open for my two younger brothers that shut for me. I hadn't yet heard the term patriarchy or been exposed to the *isms*; that revelation was to come later in my life. All I knew was that I was living in the greatest country on earth where everyone wanted to live because anything and everything was possible.

In ninth grade, I had a teacher who began to poke holes in my belief system. As I look back, I wonder if he had a personal mission to show those of us with privilege a different side of things. Whatever his purpose, for many of us it did begin to open our eyes and churn out some hard questions. He assigned us books like *The Ugly American* and *A Nation of Sheep* to read and reflect on.

As I think back on those first years of being exposed to something that jeopardized my belief system, I am still amazed at how real those beliefs felt, how disorienting it was to have them threatened, especially by a different truth, and the willingness it took to integrate them into a new way of seeing. Has it become any easier over the years? Not for me, but it is an adventure to live life without having already made up our minds.

This process of examining, reflecting, and questioning is a process that is continuously before us and one that is never done. The author F. Scott Fitzgerald reminds us, "At 18 our convictions are hills from which we look; at 45 they are caves in which we hide." When we stop examining and questioning our beliefs, we open ourselves to increasing discontent, attachment, addiction, and anger. When we hide in our caves and forget to climb hills, violence, injustice, and "othering" increase.

> This process of examining, reflecting, and questioning is a process that is continuously before us and one that is never done.

A few years ago, I was having a video conversation with my then four-year-old granddaughter Franklynn, when she inadvertently dropped the phone. She was distraught as she quickly picked up the phone and anxiously asked, "Grandma, are you okay?" "I'm fine," I replied. "But," she said, "I saw you fall!" To her four-year-old mind, I was in the phone, and I fell when the phone fell.

Like so many stories that are shared about the way small children make sense of things, we chuckle at their plausible deductions. We also expect them to grow out of it. At some point, Franklynn was able to grasp that although she could see me in the phone, I wasn't actually in it.

Phil Nuernberger, PhD, once said that in yoga, all beliefs are designed to eventually fail. He went on to say that the purpose of a belief is to take us to a larger level of understanding and, once integrated, to then be replaced by a more inclusive belief that leads us to the next level of understanding. Ultimately, we find freedom from everything, but it is a freedom without disdain, judgment, or a sense of superiority. It is a freedom that includes everything but is also beyond all things.

In the process, the inside of us is changed, and the eyes with which we look out at each other and inward at ourselves see differently. But we must be willing to actively seek to know what we don't know and to sit in confusion when our experience contradicts our belief. This process is a continuous lifelong invitation that asks us to open to the unfamiliar, hold fast to our integrity, and to be able to discern the difference.

In our society today, this is often not the case. Some of us are so adamant about the correctness of our beliefs that we attempt to cajole others into believing what we believe, even refusing contact with family members and friends who disagree with us. Yet Patanjali reminds us friendliness, compassion, happiness, and non-judgment are the highest qualities available to human nature and the resting place for peaceful minds, not fighting for our limited understanding.

But how do we know what to believe? In a world of so many contradictory beliefs, each adamantly claiming to be true, how do we stay open, steadfast, and discerning? This process is a fragile one and not one to be taken lightly. After all, there are a lot of "truths" clamoring for our attention.

We ask ourselves, "What kind of world is this belief creating?"

To help us discern, we can measure these ideas against an ethical yardstick. Does this belief promote the wellbeing of all, or just a few? Does this belief promote fear and the need for protection, or trust and the desire to share? Does this belief promote hatred and violence, or tolerance and peace? What kind of a world is this belief creating?

For yoga, the bottom line is first do no harm. This guideline requires constant vigilance over our own knowing acts of harm, and constant seeking of the places we are blind to the harm we have caused and continue to cause. Where have we unwittingly kept others, animals, the earth, from thriving? Where have we not told the truth about the land we stand on and the real cost of how we live? Nonviolence is an educational process that awakens us to the places and ways we are in need of repenting, reconciling, and repairing. It involves truth telling, respect, and reciprocity.

I remember well something the theologian John Dominic Crossan said in a lecture I attended many years ago. He was being jeered by audience members who disagreed with what he was saying. He responded with these words, which I have paraphrased, "The bottom line is, if I am the one in power, I will allow you to have your beliefs; if you are the one in power, you will persecute me for my beliefs."

It is interesting, I think, to look at the formidable challenges we face through the eyes of the *kleshas*. The actions of our limited understanding create repercussions that we can't address unless, in the words of F. Scott Fitzgerald, we are willing to climb another mountain where the view is more expansive. Nothing is solved in the caves where we cling to our small boxes of knowing.

On the morning of my son David's seventh birthday, I asked him to turn around so I could see how big he was now that he had grown a year. He smiled proudly at the accomplishment of being older, and then, for the first time, became interested in the back side of his body. I showed him how to stand with his back to a full-length mirror, hold a hand mirror just right, and see what was reflected in the mirror. On seeing himself from that angle, he giggled in delight and returned several times during the day to reaffirm what the mirror had shown him. For the first time, he was able to contact a part of himself he had never seen before, and it gave him a larger perspective and a sense of wholeness that was not previously available to him.

A few years ago, my spouse officiated the marriage of a young couple. In his sermon, he used the metaphor of "crossing the aisle." Seems this couple always sat on opposite sides of the church until one day the young man decided to switch sides and move toward the young woman. This crossing led to the eventual commitment of these two people to share their lives together in a profound and intimate way.

The image of "crossing the aisle" has stayed with me as I notice how often I tend to sit in the same chair, on the same side of my life. But to grow, we need to move. We need to cross the aisle into new perspectives, into the unfamiliar, into what seems scary, into what seems too unworthy or too magnificent.

We are beings created with infinite possibilities to expand ourselves. Each effort at expansion begins with a simple crossing of the aisle and a willingness to break out of our habitual box.

Reflection: Name one or two beliefs you currently hold that used to be hills you explored from, and have now become caves you hide in (refer to F. Scott Fitzgerald quote).

Reflection: Do something bold to "cross the aisle" into a new perspective, into the unfamiliar, into what seems scary, or into what seems too unworthy or too magnificent.

Those Who Seem Different

As I wrote this chapter, Ruth Bader Ginsberg had just died. Not long before, John Lewis had died. They were both respected for their integrity and consistency so much so that Ruth Bader Ginsberg was referred to as the soul of the Supreme Court, and John Lewis was referred to as the soul of the Senate.

I mention them now because their passing feels current and brings up again the question for me, what is it about some people that make them, for lack of a better word, great? What is it that causes others to take notice of these unique individuals? I'll admit I have always been enamored with people who seem to imbue a higher quality of humanity. Some are from history; others are alive today. Some are widely known; others hold a quieter influence. Some are found in politics, some in the healing traditions, and still others in places we might not think to look. Some I have read about; others I have met personally; others I will never know.

What is it, I wonder, about these ordinary humans that make them seem extraordinary? What is it that commands our respect and acknowledges their integrity even when we might not agree with them? What is it about them that bears witness to the fact of human possibility?

Like us, they must have felt the pull to sensory stimulation, greed, and excess; yet they seemed to stay steadfast in their focus on things greater than themselves. Like us, they endured personal loss and pain; yet they seemed to promote healing, acceptance, and forgiveness. Like us, they must have been tempted by the voices of apathy and despair; yet they displayed courage and hope.

It is as if they knew their lives could only be truly satisfied by giving, not by hoarding; by serving, not by pampering; by loving, not by needing to be loved; by something greater than themselves, not by their own petty needs. That knowledge led them from self-absorption to a love in service of a greater good.

As I reflect on these people I admire, I am astounded by how much good they accomplished. Countries were freed, hospitals built for the poor, unfair laws changed, the poor and destitute loved and cared for....the list goes on and on; suffice it to say that it seems each of them accomplished more than I could in lifetimes. And they did it from a place of seemingly limitless energy and an almost childlike joy.

When I was actively doing protesting, I went to the Nevada Test Site to do civil disobedience against the underground testing of nuclear bombs. I was excited to know that Dom Hélder Câmara would be there and would be speaking to a group of us who had gathered. Dom Hélder was a Catholic priest who, at that time, chose to live in the barrios of Brazil ministering to the poorest of the poor amongst the growing injustices of poverty. Daily, he witnessed the horror of infant death, undernourishment, disease, and extreme hardship. (Perhaps you know him from this quote, "When I feed the poor, they call me a saint, but when I ask why the poor are hungry, they call me a communist.")

I was much younger then, and, in an odd sort of way, wanted to hear him "lay into" those beliefs and systems directly responsible for such inhumanity. But he didn't do that. Instead, he got up to the podium and, as tears freely flowed from his eyes, he looked up at the sky. All he could say was, "Do you see how the stars twinkle and the sun shines?"

I am embarrassed to say at the time I was disappointed in his talk; I didn't get it. I wasn't mature enough to understand the profoundness of his words. You see, Dom Hélder Câmara had an inner landscape that had room for nothing else but wonder, mystery, and gratitude. It is said that he worked tirelessly in the barrios from 6:00 am until late at night, but every morning he arose at 2:00 am to pray for four hours before ministering to the poor. He spent four hours a day in communion with his God watering and nourishing the seeds of compassion, love, and service.

Gandhi, too, had eyes that saw the world from a generous inner self. He was the first to fully understand that the oppressor suffers as much as the oppressed. He understood the profound truth that when there is suffering, everyone suffers. What an amazing mind and heart Gandhi had, that he could see the suffering of the oppressor, and reach out, not with anger, but with the strong arm of justice mixed with compassion.

Both Dom Hélder Câmara and Mahatma Gandhi, like us today, lived in the midst of extreme injustice and suffering. And yet they acted from a place of a rich interior and a heart that was firmly in communion with a Higher Reality. And miracles happened.

I wonder, what was it like for them? Did they ask themselves, if this heart and mind were the heart and mind of the whole world, what kind of world would it be? How did they take time to nourish the seeds of love and compassion while also tending their fiery passion for justice? How did they cut the chains that bound them to selfishness so that they could freely serve others?

I don't know what makes some of us courageous and others cowardly, what makes some of us accepting and others intolerant, some of us violent and others unable to do harm, or some of us full of love and others full of hate.

I do know that some people, whatever their religion or tradition, stand apart, and in doing so they invite us to face the ugly monsters of anger and fear and greed within us as well as in our culture. They invite us to uproot the weeds of arrogance and judgment and hopelessness within us as well as in the world. They invite us to pay attention to the choices we make and the thoughts we think.

Reflection: If your heart and mind were the heart and mind of the world, what kind of world would it be?

Finding Freedom

THE PEACE

*Internal suffering has been replaced with
an internal joy that impacts how we are
in the world.*

I am aware that freedom is an experience of which I have only some conceptual knowledge mixed with experiential glimpses. Yet those glimpses have been monumental in fueling my practice and sustaining my certainty in a state other than ignorance. One particular incident stands out in its extraordinariness, both because it lasted for three days and because it was a radical departure from the way in which I know reality. I have treasured it over the years but have shared it with few.

Words fail to relay the experience because it wasn't conceptual, it just was. I came out of my meditation time, and everything had changed. My mind was quiet. The process of thinking, as I had experienced it, was gone, and with it the roaming tendencies and mental constructs. Judgments, criticisms, analysis, liking, and disliking were no longer present. Fear and anxiety were gone. What was left was awareness. Past and future blended into the present. I wasn't telling myself about things, I was just in the experience of being with life as it was. I was in an experience unlike anything I had ever known.

For three days there was nothing I needed or wanted. A constant state of equilibrium, contentment, joy, and fulfillment filled every corner of my being. I was separate yet connected to all things in a harmonious synchronicity and rhythm out of which movement flowed. There were no decisions to make or planning or list-making in the manner I was accustomed to; rather those things happened automatically as dictated by a deeper knowing. I was in sync with the greater flow of life instead of with my own personal agenda.

It was like waking up in a parallel universe, only I woke up in a parallel mind. Nothing in my life had changed, but how I encountered it had. The experience was a totally different experience of my same life. I had been given a glimpse of a mind that sees when the clutter is gone. My software had not been updated, so to speak, but an entirely different operating system had been downloaded into me.

I don't know how I ended up in this state of awareness, but I do know that I began to feel the pull back to the thinking mind and with it the mental proclivities. My quiet mind began to get noisy. Opinions, dissatisfaction, neediness, etc., gradually found their way back into my head, and as they did, I found myself back in sync with my judgments and preferences.

It reminded me of a time when one of our granddaughters stayed with us as a toddler. We live with a view to Lake Superior, which we taught her to call "big water." We often took her to a small lake to play in the "little water." That year an overdose of rain left huge puddles on the ground that we called "water that isn't supposed to be there."

Now much older, we joke with our granddaughter about the language we used with her. Yet, in an odd way that simple language explained my experience. As the thoughts re-entered my mind, they felt like they weren't supposed to be there. And the louder and more insistent they got, the more I felt like I was back in a "little mind." I had had an experience of a "big mind," and now it was no longer available. What had been an awareness of thoughts in the distance thinking themselves, was now an experience of thinking these thoughts. I had returned to processing, planning, and remembering my life rather than being in it.

How did my mind break free? And why did it get caught again? What made the mental clutter so potent that it pulled me back? I don't have answers. I had tasted something my ego could not make up, make happen, understand, or even imagine. I had been given a small glimpse of what it might mean to exist on the other side of bondage, an existence that Patanjali calls resting in essential nature. And the roaming tendencies had pulled me back to their noise.

We often toss the words enlightenment, awakened, and freedom around in a synonymous package as if we know what these words mean. But do we? I remember one of my teaching experiences where I was using these words assuming that all of us shared a common aspiration and understanding. Then one participant said, "I'm not sure I want to be enlightened; what if I don't like it?" The room fell silent; I think we were all momentarily stunned.

Since that time, I have felt a continued gratitude to that participant for her courageous honesty. Her question has had a lasting influence on my willingness to look at my illusions about enlightenment and to humbly admit their self-serving nature. I realized I wanted to be enlightened because I assumed all my problems would go away; people would admire and like me, and I could float through the rest of my life with ease and contentment. That was ego's idea, not Patanjali's.

The caterpillar doesn't know what it is like to fly; it can only imagine what it must be like from its own limited view on the ground. The only thing available to the caterpillar is to submit itself to the process of spinning a cocoon. For those of us who are still in the caterpillar stage, entangled in the *kleshas*, what can we understand about this state of freedom? What does it mean to be free?

Freedom

Freedom is undeniably precious. At great cost, armies fight to preserve their country's freedom. Under harsh conditions, families leave their homelands in search of freedom. Despite risk, people take to the streets to protest for freedom. But what does freedom mean, and who is it for? From individual freedom to carry a gun and not wear a mask, to the freedom that restrains itself for the sake of the common good, freedom is always being sought out, argued over, and hungered for.

In her book, *On Freedom: Four Songs of Care and Constraint*, author Maggie Nelson explores what freedom means in art, sex, drugs, and climate. She raises the complex question of where "anything goes" ends and care and constraint become crucial, because, as she points out, freedom is always in relation to something.

Freedom is always in relation to something.

When Patanjali uses the word freedom he uses it to describe the freedom attained when the mind has been stilled and the *kleshas* rendered impotent. This kind of freedom does not mean we can do anything we want. In fact, we may notice that Patanjali begins the path to freedom with the *yamas*, or restraints. Restraining from harm, from excess, from inauthenticity, etc., with ourselves and others is foundational to finding and maintaining ultimate freedom.

Awareness of the ways we are in bondage to the *kleshas* plus the ongoing discipline of practice reveal a "tug of war"

191

experience between bondage and the hunger for freedom. One moment we are sourced in internal wellbeing; the next moment we are saying something snarky about our neighbor. One moment we feel lovingly held by a Higher Reality; the next moment we are stuck in our selfish, small self. Yogic texts are full of stories of ongoing battles between two opposing forces that speak to this battle within us.

When Patanjali teaches about freedom, he is aware of this arduous struggle because he (and other great souls before him) have endured this struggle and emerged victorious. While we may carry distorted ideas about freedom, Patanjali has something else in mind. The word *kaivalya* that gets translated as absolute freedom in English, has the meaning of "alone," "standing on its own," "not needing anything else," "complete in itself."

When I have flashed these words on a screen while teaching, the reception is a hushed silence. I imagine others in the room are processing these words in much the same way I do, as anything but appealing to the idea our ego has of freedom. Besides sounding somewhat dull, these words sound like we don't care about anything or anyone. But is that true?

The kind of freedom described here is freedom from ignorance (*avidya*), the root cause of our suffering. Gone is our distorted thinking. Gone is the feeling of loneliness and alienation. Gone is the need to have more than anyone else or to be superior to everyone else. Gone is the internal suffering caused by doubt, fear, confusion, and disillusionment. Gone is our need to burden others with our anger or neediness.

We know what it is like to be in bondage: the constant effort to impress others, to fight with the moment or try to manipulate it. We know the ups and downs of being on top of the world one moment and in the pits the next. We may have long stretches of happiness, but always something provokes a descent to despair or at least some form of disappointment. We know what it is like to be anxious and afraid.

> To be free is to be free of the drama and conflict that often accompany us. It is to be sourced internally, in touch with that which doesn't waver.

In contrast, to be free is to be free of the drama and conflict that often accompany us. It is to be sourced internally, in touch with that which doesn't waver. Internal suffering has been replaced with an internal joy that impacts how we are in the world.

Reflection: What is freedom (economically, spiritually, physically, mentally, emotionally, politically)? Who is it for?

Reflection: In what ways do restraints and freedom go together? In other words, why do you think Patanjali began the 8-limbed path with restraints as a requirement for attaining freedom?

A Different Mind

It was clear that the treasured frescoes, painted by Michelangelo on the ceiling of the Sistine Chapel, needed attention. The ceiling bore signs of structural damage, and a thick layer of soot and grime covered the artwork above. So began the most recent restoration project, a process that occurred between 1980-1994. The team in charge of the restoration spent six months laboring over scientific studies in search of the most effective solvents and methods to use. The probing question was how could the restoration best be addressed without harming the treasured paintings underneath?

Once the team of experts settled on an approach, work on the project began. When the restoration was complete, the cracks had been fixed, the soot and grime removed, and an intensity of color flooded the chapel ceiling, bringing stunning clarity and vibrancy to Michelangelo's paintings.

> Our dedication to our practice has begun to remove the layers of soot from our mind and reveal the potency and tranquility hiding under the noise of the *kleshas*.

It is much the same with our minds. What we have become used to as normal, we now realize was damage and grime caused by the *kleshas*. Our dedication to our practice has begun to remove the layers of soot and reveal the potency and tranquility hiding under the noise of the *kleshas* and the busyness of the roaming tendencies.

The mind that was stuck roaming around thoughts of chocolate chip cookies, how much someone hurt us, how much better other people have it than we do, (insert your own litany), has been replaced with a mind ready to explore its inexhaustible potential. Freed from pettiness and roaming, the innate faculties of creating, visioning, perceiving, discovering, solving, and discerning are readily available. Our minds have been restored to their inherent tranquil nature.

Reflection: Look up pictures of the latest restoration of the Sistine Chapel. Reflect on the difference between before and after the restoration. How might these pictures serve as an image for your practice?

Reflection: What do you think your mind would be capable of if it wasn't occupied with regrets, attachments, blame, victimhood, and whatever various ways you damper your own mind's potential?

A Different Identity

When the mind has become still, we no longer know ourselves as the fluctuating contents of our minds (the fundamental mistake of *avidya*—ignorance of who we are); we now know ourselves as we truly are (essential nature, true nature, consciousness, spirit, Buddha nature, and Christ consciousness are some of the names for this experience). This is not something we've become; it's who we were all along. This is who we were before the world told us about ourselves. Our fluctuating identity is now a stable identity, a constant sense of contentment and fulfillment grounded in an unchanging Higher Reality.

> When the mind has become still, we know ourselves as we truly are. This is our essential nature. This is not something we've become; it's who we were all along. This is who we were before the world told us about ourselves.

What is our essential nature like? We can't really know until we experience it ourselves. But the mystics of all faith traditions give us glimpses. They seem to have taken up permanent residence in their essential nature; perhaps that is why we feel drawn to them. Transported to a realm of joy and love, no matter what their momentary hardships, difficulties, or misfortunes, to them, everything is nourishment for the soul.

They seem to rest in a sea of benevolence, nourishment, and magnanimity. Their poetry and metaphor invite us to taste, see, and smell this essence of wellbeing. Because they are identified with this essence, they embody the same qualities, and give us a flavor of our true selves.

When we seek to know who we are and what can be revealed when the mind is our friend, life gets turned upside down, or maybe I should say right side up. As we become more centered, we paradoxically realize we are not the center. Rather than hoard and protect for the future, we instead serve the future. Rather than take pleasure in personal excess, we take pleasure in balance and reciprocity. Rather than build strength by force, we build strength in vulnerability. Our greed has become generosity, our selfishness has become service, and our fear has become love.

Nothing has changed; everything has changed. The yoga masters describe this as being in the world but not of it. The world is the same, but we are no longer caterpillars. We have become butterflies.

When my grandchildren were small, I would hold them and walk to a mirror. Their eyes would light up as they immediately recognized grandma in the mirror, but they had no idea who it was that grandma was holding. Each time I would point to their image in the mirror and say their name. Even so, it took time and repeated visits to the mirror for them to begin to recognize themselves as the one grandma was holding. I remember the moment they looked in the mirror and finally, giggling with delight, knew they were seeing themselves. And with that recognition, they knew what they looked like.

Like these small children, we too, are in the process of recognizing our true selves.

Reflection: Who are you when all the roles, adjectives, and ways of knowing yourself are taken away?

Reflection: What are some of the qualities of a person who "rests in their essential nature"?

Grace

Through the sustained effort of practice and nonattachment, we can soften the grip of conditioning. We can gain a more peaceful mind, a more generous heart, and a more joyful appreciation for our lives. But is this all there is to it? If we just practice, can we remove the fundamental misunderstanding of who we are? Can we make enlightenment happen on cue? Not any more than a farmer can make a seed grow. The farmer can till and prepare the soil, plant the seeds at the appropriate time, depth, and distance. The farmer can diligently tend and maintain a fertile environment for the best possible harvest. But the farmer cannot control the weather or an influx of insects or other unknowns. Nor can the farmer make the small seed sprout.

It is the same with us. We can be diligent in our practice, creating and maintaining an environment where awakening and freedom can happen. We can spin our cocoons, so to speak. But we can't turn ourselves into butterflies. We can't plan the timing; we can only trust the process and surrender to it.

There is a Higher Reality beyond the *kleshas*. It is this reality that reaches across the gulf of ignorance and lovingly carries us from lives of bondage to lives of freedom. We call this grace. And we come to realize that the desire to practice, as well as the attention to practice, is all part of grace. Higher Reality has been with us all along showering us with benevolence and compassion, gently and lovingly waking us up from bondage. (Note: Yoga believes in a Higher Reality, but it is not a religion. It is a science based on a proven, time-tested methodology. One can be a Christian, a Muslim, etc. and still be a practicing yogi.)

Perhaps if we can remember nothing else, the importance of remembering that none of us see clearly, could make our world a very different place. Perhaps we would stop being so sure of ourselves and realize that how we are seeing our world, the Higher Reality, ourselves, and each other is a projection of our own limited conditioning. Perhaps this would be enough to keep our world more peaceful and our hearts a little kinder.

> Remembering that none of us see clearly could be enough to keep our world more peaceful and our hearts a little kinder.

If we realized the wealth of possibility ready to be unlocked in our own mind, perhaps our attention would go to supporting the process that gives us access to this treasure. We can settle for a life lived within the limits of our unexamined conditioning. But there is so much more! Our minds are longing to be quieted; our inner world is there to be explored. An indescribable treasure of joy is waiting for us.

We are made to be happy. We are made to long for more. But what is happiness? And what is the "more" we long for? Our conditioning points us in one direction; a spiritual practice in another. One brings us momentary pleasures and makes us dependent on the outside world. The other promises us a lasting joy and contentment in both worlds.

How will we answer this hunger for more inside of us? With more possessions? With success? Achievement? Fame? Or will we answer it with the discipline of self-study and quiet reflection and a practice that leads us to the treasures of a quiet mind and the experience of our full selves? The choice is ours.

Reflection: What is your experience of grace?

Reflection: Ponder these words by Dr. David Frawley, "Human life is nothing but a struggle to learn to control the mind. If we have accomplished this, we have done everything and accomplished the most difficult thing in the entire universe" (Frawley, p. 55). Do you agree with Dr. David Frawley's statement? Why or why not?

Closing Thoughts

I enjoy watching movies with superheroes and heroines. No matter how desperate things get, nothing is required of me. Someone with superpowers will come along and save me, along with the rest of the planet, and take care of the bad guys. All ends well, and I haven't had to participate in my own salvation.

The conditioning that has shaped me and many others like me is funny that way. We seem to feel like we should have outcomes without much effort. We seem to love knowledge and knowing about things but like to skip over the work of experiencing them for ourselves. And although many of us feel rushed, we don't seem to feel a need or urgency for the things that really matter...perhaps because we are used to last minute rescues by superheroes.

Although I began this book many times, writing a few words here and there, the ability to maintain a sustained effort kept losing momentum as various other activities vied for my attention. The bulk of the writing and completion of this book happened in the two years that paralleled a turn in my life when I took a bad fall on the Superior Hiking Trail. Suddenly, instead of being an able-bodied person, I had a broken arm and a broken foot. Instead of flying to various parts of the country to teach, I was bound to my home. Instead of being able to care for myself, I needed vast amounts of help. It was a shocking turn of events to my whole way of knowing myself.

When I wasn't managing the pain and discomfort, I was nursing lavish thoughts of pity on myself. When I couldn't even take a walk or drive anywhere, I entertained thoughts of escape like sugary treats, alcohol, or endless television. As tempting as that immediate pleasure seemed, the long-term effects didn't look promising.

I decided to write. Even that proved difficult. In the beginning, I couldn't manage a book or a computer, but I could make some marks on paper. I started there. As things healed, I could manage to do some reading and research and even type with one finger. Over time, I could use one finger on both hands. As the casts were removed, I became mobile on my feet and had the use of all ten fingers.

But it didn't happen automatically. For decades my fingers had been gripping, grasping, twisting, playing piano, typing letters on a keyboard, peeling carrots, folding laundry, and squeezing toothpaste tubes. I thought once the cast was removed, everything would go back to normal, but my arm and fingers had forgotten how to do all these things. Furthermore, the strength in my arm and fingers had rapidly deteriorated from nonuse. Off to occupational therapy I went to be instructed on how to get back the dexterity and strength that once seemed so automatic. Now it was up to me to commit to the practice of doing the exercises. It was up to me to stay faithful through the advancements, setbacks, and plateaus.

I share this because the process itself taught me so much about the subject of this book. Bondage to the *kleshas* is like having our mind in a cast, except that the cast on our mind is invisible which makes it more insidious. I knew my arm and foot were both in a cast and my ability had been greatly compromised. Because the conditioning of *kleshas* is invisible, our mind seems "normal," and the normalcy makes it more difficult to recognize how much our minds have been compromised.

There are no superheroes who can rescue us from our distracted, scattered, foggy, fearful, anxious minds. This is the responsibility of each one of us. But we do have guidance and support in the same way that I had a surgeon who put my broken bone back together and an occupational therapist who taught me the exercises to help my arm and fingers remember what they already knew.

We have great souls who have mastered their minds and tell us of the paradise that awaits us. We have great teachers who, in their compassion, lay out the detailed path for us of the work ahead. We have spiritual centers in which to practice and like-minded people to practice with. And we have the grace of Higher Reality blessing us every step of the way. But the work, the effort, the discipline, and the choice belong to us.

There is more to reality than we know or understand.
There is more to life than getting what we want.
There is more to us than adjectives and roles.

Life can be more harmonious and satisfying,
Filled with contentment and peace of mind.
We can know who we are without having to
Describe ourselves to ourselves.

But it does take discipline,
And attending to little things,
That don't seem to matter in the moment,
That can easily be dismissed.
"What harm can this do?"
"What good will that do?" we say.

Yet we fail our own wellbeing
When we underestimate their significance.

Reflecting on our thoughts and actions,
Examining the words and ideas we react to,
Sitting quietly with ourselves,
Breathing deep into our belly,
Cultivating a grateful heart,
Being kind....
All point the mind toward freedom.

Loosening the chains that bind us is a gradual process,
and,
Even a little effort never goes to waste.

~ Deborah Adele

Acknowledgments

Endless gratitude to Panditji (Pandit Rajmani Tigunait) and the Himalayan Institute faculty, staff, and community of practitioners. This is the tradition and the people that nourish, teach, hold, and inspire my knowledge and practice.

Gratitude to past teachers who began putting cracks in my narrative. David Wolfe, Greta Gaard, Tineke Ritmeester, Carolyn Pressler, Narvada Puri, and Yogiraj Achala, you changed how I see things.

There are those who supported, held, and encouraged the writing of this book. Roger Sams, David Bowers, Sandra Bergsten, Patti Peters, Doug Dirks, Frank von Poppen, Duane Kimball, David Kimball, and Doug Paulson, your belief in me and in this book were indispensable.

A special note of gratitude to Sarah Hutchinson, Darcy Cunningham, and Sally Burgess who gave this manuscript a thorough read and improved it with invaluable comments. Your attending of time and support to this effort was an act of love.

Gratitude to Sara Duke and David Devere, without whom, for many reasons, this book would not be in print.

To those of you not mentioned by name who have and do walk with me in small and large ways, you are in this book because you shape me with your love and companionship.

And to life itself, this remarkable gift that allows for exploration, choice, expansion, learning, and joy. I am grateful for all of it.

Sources

WORKS CITED:

Taimni, I.K. *The Science of Yoga.* This material was reproduced by permission of Quest Books, imprint of The Theosophical Publishing House, www.questbooks.net, ©2005.

Tigunait, Pandit Rajmani. *The Secret of the Yoga Sutra: Samadhi Pada.* This material was reproduced by permission of Himalayan International Institute of Yoga Science & Philosophy, U.S.A., ©2014.

Frawley, David. *Ayurveda and the Mind: The Healing of Consciousness.* Reprinted with permission by Lotus Press, PO Box 325, Twin Lakes WI 53181, www.lotuspress.com, ©1997.

Sophia, Jett. *Signal Fire* #132, ©April 11, 2012. Re-released in *Signal Fire* #357, ©January 20, 2022, www.jettsophia.com.

Wiest, Brianna. "This Is What 'Self-Care' REALLY Means, Because It's Not All Salt Baths And Chocolate Cake." *Thought Catalog.* May 17, 2022. https://thoughtcatalog.com/brianna-wiest/2017/11/this-is-what-self-care-really-means-because-its-not-all-salt-baths-and-chocolate-cake/

ADDITIONAL WORKS CONSULTED:

The Practice of the Yoga Sutra: Sadhana Pada, Pandit Rajmani Tigunait, Ph.D.

The Yoga Sutras of Patanjali, Edwin F. Bryant.

Yoga Sutra Workbook: The Certainty of Freedom, Vyaas Houston, M.A.

Yogasutra Patanjali: With the Commentary of Vyasa, Bangali Baba.

About the Author

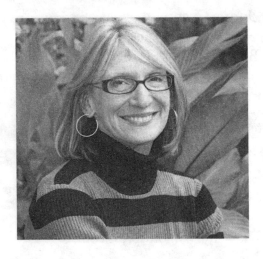

Deborah Adele holds master's degrees in both Liberal Studies and Theology & Religious Studies. She carries yoga certifications in Kundalini yoga, Hatha yoga, Yoga Therapy, and Meditation. She is also trained in Gestalt Theory and Somatic Education. From 1999-2012, Deborah brought her combined knowledge of business and her in-depth knowledge of yoga philosophy to build Yoga North, a center that continues to flourish.

In 2009 she published *The Yamas & Niyamas: Exploring Yoga's Ethical Practice*, which has become an international best-seller and a modern classic. It is a go-to book for any serious yogi and for anyone seeking deeper understanding of self.

Deborah's writing and teaching leave participants with a dynamic combination of hope, inspiration, and practical knowledge.

Visit Deborah at www.DeborahAdele.com.